I0845746

Sleeve Gastrectomy Surgery Unleashed

Your Witty Q&A Guide to Slimming Success

Jihad Kudsi, MD

Sleeve Gastrectomy Surgery Unleashed

Your Witty Q&A Guide to Slimming Success

Copyright © 2023 Jihad Kudsi, MD

First Edition

All rights reserved.

The content of this book, including text, images, and illustrations, is protected by copyright law. Unauthorized use, reproduction, or distribution of any part of this book is strictly prohibited without prior written permission from the copyright owner. Infringement may result in legal action.

Legal Disclaimer

The information provided in this book is for general informational purposes only and is not a substitute for professional medical advice. Always consult a qualified healthcare provider for medical guidance. The authors and publishers are not liable for any errors or omissions or any consequences from using the information in this book. Mention of medical procedures, products, or opinions does not constitute an endorsement. Reliance on the book's content is at your own risk. This disclaimer is subject to change and was last updated on 8/9/2023.

Jihad Kudsi, MD

8/9/2023

Dedication

To my wife, Diala, and my daughters, Layla and Naya,

This dedication is a tribute to the incredible love and unwavering support you have bestowed upon me. Diala, your presence by my side has been my anchor, providing strength and encouragement in every endeavor. Layla and Naya, your innocent smiles and boundless joy remind me of the beauty and wonder in life.

To Dergham and Maha, my remarkable parents,

Your unwavering support, belief, and guidance have shaped me into the person I am today. You have instilled in me the values of resilience, love, and determination that have fueled my journey. This dedication is a testament to your profound influence on my life.

To Dina, Zaki, Bana, and Hassan, my beloved siblings,

Your love, camaraderie, and shared experiences have enriched my life beyond measure. Through laughter and challenges, we have grown together, forming an unbreakable bond. This dedication extends to each of you, as you each have played an integral role in my journey.

With heartfelt gratitude and love,

Jihad Kudsi

7/5/2023

Contents

Introduction

Welcome to Sleeve Gastrectomy Surgery Unleashed: Your Witty Q&A Guide to Slimming Success, a book designed to accompany and empower you on your remarkable journey toward a healthier and happier life.

I'm Dr. Jihad Kudsi – a bariatric surgeon on a mission to change lives through weight loss and better health. With extensive experience in minimally invasive surgery, including sleeve gastrectomy, gastric bypass, and more, I've helped countless individuals achieve their wellness goals. I am double board-certified in General Surgery and Obesity Medicine and fellowship trained in bariatric surgery, I'm all about providing comprehensive care with compassion and dedication. Let's work together to transform your life for the better!

In a world where countless weight loss methods and fad diets promise quick fixes and magical transformations, sleeve gastrectomy surgery has proven to be a powerful tool that has revolutionized the lives of many individuals seeking long-term weight loss success. However, embarking on such a journey can be overwhelming, filled with questions, doubts, and uncertainties.

That's where this book comes in. This is a unique resource that not only provides you with comprehensive information about sleeve gastrectomy surgery but also presents it in an engaging and witty question-and-answer format. The goal is to equip you with knowledge, insights, and practical tips to navigate this transformative process with confidence and clarity.

In these pages, you will find answers to the most commonly asked questions about sleeve gastrectomy surgery, ranging from the procedure itself to post-operative care, lifestyle changes, and the emotional aspects of the journey. The book takes a lighthearted approach, infusing humor and relatability into the answers to keep you engaged and motivated throughout your reading experience.

But this book goes beyond mere information. It aims to address not just the physical aspects of slimming success but also the emotional and psychological factors that are often intertwined with our relationship with food and self-image.

Whether you are contemplating sleeve gastrectomy surgery, have recently undergone the procedure, or are in the process of post-operative recovery, this book is tailored to meet your needs. It is meant to guide you, inspire you, and remind you that you are not alone on this journey.

So, dear reader, let this book be your trusted companion, your source of knowledge, and your cheerleader as you navigate the ups and downs of your slimming success journey. Embrace the wit, wisdom, and encouragement found within these pages, and embark on a transformation that will redefine your relationship with yourself and the world around you.

Together, let us embrace sleeve gastrectomy surgery as a powerful tool for change, and let us uncover the secrets to lasting, sustainable, and joyful slimming success. The journey starts now.

1. The biggest question: What is sleeve gastrectomy?

Okay, so you are wondering about sleeve gastrectomy! Basically, this surgery modifies your stomach to make it smaller, like a sleeve. Hence the name, sleeve gastrectomy —makes sense, right? During the procedure, the surgeon takes out a big chunk of your stomach, leaving behind a tube-shaped, banana-like stomach. This new stomach limits how much food you can eat at one time. It's like shrinking the space, so you literally can't overeat anymore. Plus, it messes with the hormones that control your hunger and appetite. We remove the part of the stomach that makes those hormones, so you feel less hungry and don't get as many cravings. And voila! It's easier to choose healthier foods and drop those pounds. Pretty neat, huh?

Sleeve gastrectomy

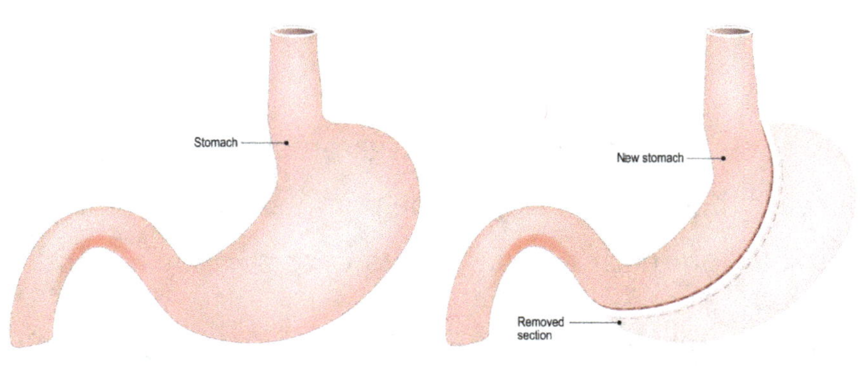

5

2. How does sleeve gastrectomy work?

So, here's the deal with sleeve gastrectomy, my friend. It basically does two things to help you shed those pounds: restricts your eating and impacts your hormones a bit.

First, let's discuss restriction. When your surgeon takes out a chunk of your stomach, obviously, it becomes smaller. So, when you eat, you will feel full faster. Say goodbye to those bottomless pit feelings! With a smaller stomach, you naturally eat fewer calories. Just like you can't fit as much water in juice glass as a Yeti tumbler, your stomach will now be satisfied more quickly!

Then there are the hormonal changes. Turns out, that chunk of stomach your surgeon will remove produces a hormone called ghrelin. Ghrelin is like the "hunger hormone"—it tells your brain you feel hungry. But a sleeve gastrectomy reduces the production of ghrelin, so your brain is not being told you are hungry as often. This makes it easier for you to control your food intake and develop healthier eating habits. So, when you combine these restrictions and hormonal changes, you're on your way to losing a bunch of weight. But remember, sleeve gastrectomy isn't some quick fix or an easy way out. It's a tool that, along with good food choices, exercise, and support, can help you lose weight and get healthier!

3. Who is a good candidate for sleeve gastrectomy?

Alright, let's dive into the qualifications for this weight-loss wonder surgery known as sleeve gastrectomy. But hey, not everyone gets a golden ticket to this stomach-shrinking extravaganza. Here's what makes a person a prime candidate for sleeve gastrectomy:

1. BMI – We're talking about Body Mass Index, folks. It's like a math equation for your health, calculating your height and weight to determine if you're in the obesity zone. Most of the time, if your BMI hits 35 or higher, it's sleeve gastrectomy time! But wait, there's more! If your BMI is between 30 and 35 and you also have medical issues caused by your excess weight, like diabetes, high blood pressure, or sleep apnea, then surgery might also be the answer to your weighty woes. You can check your BMI on my website DoctorKudsi.com.

2. Failed Attempts at Weight Loss – You must show some effort, people! If you've already tried diets and intense

workouts but couldn't keep the pounds off for the long haul, then you're a potential star candidate. Sleeve gastrectomy is for those who've battled the bulge and need some serious backup.

3. Health Problems Galore – It's like a two-for-one deal! Sleeve gastrectomy not only helps you shed pounds but also can fix those pesky health problems caused by your larger physique. If you're dealing with type 2 diabetes, high blood pressure, sleep apnea, or joint pain, then this surgery might be your saving grace. Say goodbye to those troubles and hello to a healthier, happier you!

4. Lifestyle Commitment – Listen up, folks, this isn't a magic wand that will zap away your extra weight while you lounge on the couch. Sleeve gastrectomy requires dedication and a serious lifestyle makeover. You must be ready to revamp your eating habits, embrace regular exercise, and follow your healthcare team's instructions post-surgery. It's like signing up for a weight-loss boot camp, but with a smaller stomach. If you're up for the challenge, then sleeve

gastrectomy can be your secret weapon for long-term success.

5. Mental Mojo – It's not just about your physical state. It's about your mental readiness, too. Before jumping into the surgery, you'll need a psychological evaluation to ensure you're mentally and emotionally prepared. Having realistic goals, understanding the risks and benefits, and being ready to embrace the physical and mental changes are key. So, buckle up, buttercup, because this journey requires a strong mindset.

6. Age and Overall Health – Age is just a number, my friends. But your overall health does matter. The surgical team will give you the once-over to ensure you're fit for the procedure. Expect some tests to make sure you're good to go and can handle the sleeve gastrectomy safely.

7. Follow-Up Frenzy – Brace yourself for some post-surgery love. If you're in the sleeve gastrectomy club, be prepared for long-term follow-ups with your healthcare team. These meetings are like checkpoints on your weight-loss journey, making sure you're on

track, addressing concerns, and setting you up for long-term success. Remember, you're not alone in this journey. Embrace the support system your healthcare team offers and commit to those follow-ups for a winning outcome.

So, there you have it, the criteria for becoming a sleeve gastrectomy VIP. If you meet these qualifications, you're likely ready to embark on a weight-loss adventure like no other. It's time to say goodbye to the old you and welcome the even more fabulous, slimmer version of you with open arms!

4. What are the benefits of sleeve gastrectomy?

Sleeve gastrectomy, aka the stomach shrinker! It's a surgical procedure that helps folks battling obesity in some seriously cool ways. Check out these benefits:

Significant Weight Loss: With sleeve gastrectomy, you can shed a whopping 30% of your weight, and some lucky ducks even lose up to 50% of their body mass. How does it work? Well, your surgeon will make your stomach smaller, so you can't devour as much food in one sitting. It's like a built-in portion control system, helping you cut calories and achieve that slow and steady weight loss. And hey, those hormonal changes will also come to your rescue, curbing those pesky cravings. Say goodbye to those extra pounds and hello to a healthier you!

Long-term Weight Loss: Forget yo-yo dieting! Sleeve gastrectomy gives you the power to control your weight for the long haul. Your appetite takes a chill pill, and smaller portions make you feel full. It's like having a personal portion police to keep you on track. So, wave goodbye to those days of mindless snacking and embrace a healthier eating routine. It's a game-changer!

Improved Health Conditions: The perks keep piling up! When you're overweight, your health can take a serious hit, with problems like diabetes, high blood pressure, sleep apnea, and joint pain creeping in. But fear not, sleeve gastrectomy can be your superhero. It can work wonders in improving or even vanquishing these pesky health issues. For many, as the pounds melt away, so does the need for excessive medications. It's like hitting the reset button on your health and giving those problems a swift kick to the curb!

Better Quality of Life: Who says life can't be fabulous? Being overweight can put a damper on your physical, mental, and social wellbeing. But fear not, the sleeve gastrectomy squad is here to save the day! With the extra weight gone, you'll find yourself doing things you never thought possible. Hello, new hobbies and active adventures! Plus, your confidence levels will skyrocket, leading to better emotional health and stronger relationships. Get ready for a life upgrade.

Longevity Bonus: Here's the real deal, my friends. Obesity is linked to some seriously scary stuff like heart disease, stroke, cancer, and other long-term illnesses. But guess what? Sleeve gastrectomy is your secret weapon against these villains. The weight loss you'll experience after surgery dramatically reduces your risk of developing these life-threatening conditions, giving you the keys to a longer, happier life. Studies even suggest that it can add 5 to 10 extra years to your glorious journey. Talk about a life-extending makeover!

Boosted Mental and Emotional Health: Prepare for a mind-blowing transformation! When you lose weight through sleeve gastrectomy, your mental and emotional wellbeing get a serious upgrade. Imagine having increased self-confidence, a brand-new body image, and an overall self-esteem boost. Sayonara, negative vibes! You'll be waving goodbye to depression and anxiety and saying hello to improved mental health, stronger relationships, and killer social interactions. Get ready to shine!

Fewer Medications, More Moolah: Wallet rejoice! As the pounds melt away and your health improves, you'll find yourself needing fewer medications. That's right, it's a double win! Your body is thriving, and your wallet is dancing a happy dance. You'll have more moolah for the fun stuff in life. Who knew losing weight could be so financially rewarding?

5. How much weight can I expect to lose after sleeve gastrectomy?

Alright, hold on tight and get ready for some weight-loss math that will make your excess pounds shake in their boots!

Let's break it down: After the surgery, you have a chance to bid farewell to that excess weight that's been dragging you down. On average, you can expect to lose a whopping 50% to 70% of that extra baggage within the first two years. So, if you're lugging around 100 pounds of extra weight, you could potentially kiss around 50 to 70 pounds goodbye!

But wait, there's more! Unlike in a thrilling game of weight loss roulette, the outcome isn't solely determined by luck. Nope, a mix of factors come into play. Your starting weight sets the stage for the grand performance. Then, it's all about sticking to those post-surgery lifestyle changes. And let's not forget about your individual metabolism, which can be as unique as a fingerprint. All of these factors work together to determine how much weight you'll actually lose.

So, remember, the numbers may vary from person to person, but with determination, a pinch of humor, and a layer of lifestyle changes, you'll be shedding those pounds in no time. Ready, set, weight-loss!

6. Can sleeve gastrectomy help with high blood pressure?

Many who struggle with obesity also have high blood pressure, which can lead to all sorts of issues. But fear not, my friend, because sleeve gastrectomy might just be what we need to bring those blood pressure readings down to earth!

You see, excess weight can be like a mischievous little imp that messes with your blood pressure. But sleeve gastrectomy takes that imp and gives it a one-way ticket out of town! As the pounds melt away, your blood pressure might just follow suit.

But wait, there's more! I'm sure you know by now sleeve gastrectomy also has an incredible impact on your body's hormones. These hormone changes can help regulate the intricate dance of your cardiovascular system.

Now, the time it takes for your blood pressure to adjust can vary from person to person, but many individuals start seeing improvements within a few weeks to a few months after the surgery. And that's why checking your blood pressure regularly is super important! It helps you and your healthcare team keep track of how well things are progressing and ensure you're on the right track. This way, they can make any necessary adjustments to your treatment plan if needed.

Lowering your blood pressure has some awesome benefits. It can significantly reduce the risk of heart disease, stroke, and other cardiovascular issues. Plus, you'll likely feel more energetic and have an improved overall sense of well-being.

Now, keep in mind that each person's journey is unique. High blood pressure can have various underlying causes, and sleeve gastrectomy might not be the perfect solution for everyone's blood pressure issues.

7. Can sleeve gastrectomy help with type 2 diabetes?

Don't get too attached to your blood sugar monitor because we're about to explore how sleeve gastrectomy can impact type 2 diabetes!

Here's the scoop: Sleeve gastrectomy works its magic by reducing the size of your stomach, making you feel full faster. But that's not all! This reduction in stomach size also leads to changes in gut hormones (glucagon-like peptide-1 [GLP-1], for example). These gut hormones play a crucial role in regulating your blood sugar levels and how your body handles insulin. So, when you undergo sleeve gastrectomy, the gut hormones become supercharged, working overtime to keep your blood sugar in check.

Now, can sleeve gastrectomy make diabetes go away completely? Well, in some cases, especially for those with type 2 diabetes, the surgery has been known to lead to remission. That means their blood sugar levels improve so much that they might not need diabetes medication anymore. It's like a "goodbye" to diabetes for some lucky ones!

But keep in mind, it's not a guarantee for everyone. For those who are insulin-dependent, the surgery might not entirely replace the need for insulin. However, it can still be a game-changer. It can often reduce the amount of insulin needed, making management a lot easier and improving overall health.

So overall your body become more sensitive to insulin, making it easier to keep your blood sugar levels steady. Some folks see improvements pretty quickly, while for others, it might take a few months or longer. Patience is key! So please don't immediately toss your blood sugar monitor away. It's still important to stay vigilant, work closely with your healthcare team, especially in the first few weeks after surgery, and follow their guidance to ensure optimal diabetes management.

8. Can sleeve gastrectomy help with sleep apnea?

Picture this: You're lying in bed, trying to catch some Z's, when suddenly your snoring reaches rock concert levels. It's not just a regular snore, it's a symphony of sawing logs that can wake up the entire neighborhood! But then, suddenly, there's complete silence, followed by a huge wheeze. That, my friend, is sleep apnea—a condition where your breathing gets interrupted during sleep, leaving you gasping for air like a fish out of water.

Now when you undergo sleeve gastrectomy, your stomach gets smaller, and your food intake takes a nosedive. But what's the connection between a smaller stomach and sleep apnea, you ask? Well, grab your popcorn, because here's the plot twist!

Excess weight can be a sneaky villain that contributes to sleep apnea. It puts pressure on your airways, making it harder for air to flow freely and causing those pesky breathing interruptions. But fear not, for sleeve gastrectomy swoops in like a mighty avenger and helps you shed those pounds!

As you lose weight after the surgery, the pressure on your airways decreases. It opens up the blocked tunnels, allowing air to flow as smoothly as if you're standing in a gentle breeze on a summer's day. No more gasping for breath like a goldfish in distress!

However, keep in mind that sleeve gastrectomy might not be the perfect solution for everyone. Sleep apnea has various causes, and weight loss surgery is just one piece of the puzzle. It's always best to consult with your doctor to determine the best course of action for your specific situation.

9. Can sleeve gastrectomy help with acid reflux or GERD?

Well, well, well, let's investigate whether sleeve gastrectomy can tame the fiery beast known as acid reflux or GERD. This topic is so important its worth discussing few times, so bear with me!

Here's the scoop: If you're grappling with GERD, there's good news and a bit of a coin toss. It's like flipping a pancake and seeing if it lands with a smiley face or a frowny face. Studies show that there's roughly a 50/50 chance that your GERD symptoms will improve after sleeve gastrectomy. Which means there is also a 50/50 change your GERD symptoms might stay the same or even get worse!

As you bid farewell to those excess pounds and your stomach undergoes a transformation, you might find that the flames of acid reflux dim and the discomfort ease. It's like a magic trick that leaves you saying, "Abracadabra, GERD be gone!"

But, here's a juicy tidbit: If you're on a quest for maximum GERD improvement, you might want to consider the heavyweight champion of weight loss surgery—gastric bypass! It's like trading in your small candle for a flamethrower to battle GERD. Gastric bypass has shown a higher success rate in relieving GERD symptoms compared to sleeve gastrectomy. It's like going from a cozy bonfire to an all-out fireworks extravaganza of GERD relief! More about gastric bypass later!

Now, let's imagine a scenario where you've chosen the sleeve gastrectomy, but unfortunately, your worst nightmare becomes a reality—your GERD is no longer under control, despite all the antacids in the world. But fear not, my friend, because you haven't burned any bridges just yet. There's still another option on the table: the mighty gastric bypass, ready to tackle both more weight loss and the quest to conquer your GERD.

Any revisional surgery is no walk in the park though, so it's time to weigh your options wisely. Choosing between surgeries can be as complex as untangling a ball of yarn while blindfolded. Remember, my friend, your journey is unique, and what works for someone else may not be the perfect fit for you. That's why it's crucial to have that in-person discussion with your surgeon and to come armed with a list of questions!

10. Can sleeve gastrectomy help with emotional eating or binge eating disorder?

Ah, the tangled web of emotions and eating! Let's work on unraveling this.

For countless individuals facing weight challenges, the journey involves more than just physical aspects—it often delves into the realm of emotions. The sleeve gastrectomy, while not a panacea for all emotional struggles, can play a pivotal role in addressing emotional eating.

You see, my friend, the sleeve gastrectomy works its magic by reducing the size of your stomach, putting a limit on the amount of food you can devour in one sitting. It's like having a bouncer at the entrance of your stomach, checking IDs and saying, "Sorry, no more room for excessive binging!"

But here's the thing: emotional eating and binge eating are cunning foes. They have a way of sneaking back into our lives, trying to crash the party like unwanted guests. That's where the sleeve gastrectomy comes in! It helps by providing a tool that empowers you to take control of your eating habits.

Now, combine that tool with some good old self-awareness and emotional intelligence, and you've got yourself a powerful duo. By being mindful of your emotions and developing healthier coping mechanisms, you'll be ready to conquer those emotional eating gremlins and binge eating dragons like a boss!

But let's not forget the importance of a support network. Surround yourself with cheerleaders who have your back, whether it's friends, family, or even an official support group. They'll be there to provide laughter, encouragement, and a gentle nudge when needed. Also remember when you saw that awesome psychiatrist or therapist before your surgery for the all-important preoperative clearance? Well, guess what? They're not just there to check boxes and give you the thumbs up! They're part of your post-op recovery too, ready to swoop in with their superpowers of support and guidance. Having a therapist in your corner can be a game-changer, and here's why:

They're the ultimate emotional support coach: Let's face it, emotions can be as unpredictable as a squirrel on a sugar rush. After surgery, you might find yourself navigating a whole new range of emotions. A therapist can help you make sense of those emotions, offering guidance and providing tools to deal with any emotional bumps in the road.

They're like a "brain mechanic." Your mind is a complex engine, my friend, and sometimes it needs a tune-up. A therapist can help you work through any mental roadblocks, self-doubts, or negative thoughts that might pop up. Think of it as a mental oil change that keeps your engine running smoothly.

They're the masters of self-discovery: Post-surgery is a time of transformation, not just physically but mentally as well. A therapist can help you explore your new identity, reframe your relationship with food, and navigate body image challenges with grace and maybe a little humor!

They're the voice of reason: Let's be real, we all have those moments when we need someone to slap us with a reality check. A therapist can gently nudge you back on track and help you challenge unhelpful thoughts.

They're your accountability partner: Remember that slice of cake you devoured in one sitting? Well, a therapist can help you stay accountable to your goals, gently reminding you of your commitment to a healthier lifestyle.

So, my fellow post-surgery explorer, while a therapist isn't mandatory, they can be an invaluable addition to your support team. They'll provide you with tools and insights to navigate the ups and downs of your sleeve gastrectomy journey.

11. Can sleeve gastrectomy help with polycystic ovary syndrome (PCOS)?

The relationship between PCOS and obesity can be described as a two-way street. PCOS and obesity can influence each other, creating a complex interplay between the two.

On one hand, PCOS can contribute to weight gain and obesity due to hormonal imbalances. Women with PCOS often have higher levels of androgens (male hormones) and insulin resistance, which can lead to increased fat storage, especially in the abdominal area. Additionally, PCOS may cause difficulties in managing weight due to metabolic and hormonal irregularities.

On the other hand, obesity can exacerbate PCOS symptoms. Adipose tissue (fat cells) can produce more androgens, leading to further hormone imbalances. This can worsen the symptoms of PCOS, such as irregular menstrual cycles, difficulty conceiving, acne, and excessive hair growth (hirsutism). But fear not, because sleeve gastrectomy might just be the solution to the PCOS problem.

When you undergo sleeve gastrectomy, it's like a hormonal power surge coursing through your body, shocking any imbalances. The weight loss that follows can have a positive impact on PCOS symptoms. It's like kicking those hormonal imbalances to the curb and telling irregular periods, "Not today, my friend!"

As you shed those extra pounds, your body's insulin starts playing nice with your cells again. This can lead to better hormone regulation, enhanced fertility, and even a reduction in those bothersome cysts on your ovaries. Sleeve gastrectomy can also help with managing other PCOS-related issues like high blood pressure, high cholesterol, and type 2 diabetes. It can be an all-in-one solution!

And just so you know, not every woman with PCOS will see the same results after the surgery. Sleeve gastrectomy isn't a guaranteed cure for PCOS. It's more like one piece of the puzzle. Dealing with PCOS is more complex, and it might involve other things like using hormone therapy.

12. Can sleeve gastrectomy improve fertility?

The question on many people's minds: Can a sleeve gastrectomy give a boost to baby-making powers?

Obesity can have a real impact on fertility, both for men and women. Here's the deal:

For women, carrying extra weight can mess with hormone levels, causing irregular periods and ovulation issues. Plus, it can lead to insulin resistance, making it harder for eggs to mature properly. That means it might take longer to get pregnant, or in some cases, it can even lead to difficulties conceiving.

And bros, it's not just the ladies – obesity can mess with men's fertility too. When guys are overweight, it can lower testosterone levels and affect sperm quality and count. So, it might take more time for them to get their partner pregnant.

Now, about sleeve gastrectomy – it can totally help both men and women! The surgery helps with weight loss by shrinking the stomach, and more importantly by changing the hormones. As a result, many peeps see significant improvements in their weight, and that can have a positive impact on fertility.

For women, losing weight after sleeve gastrectomy can regulate their menstrual cycles and make it easier to conceive. It might also improve their overall hormone levels and increase the chances of getting pregnant.

And guys, listen up – weight loss from sleeve gastrectomy can boost testosterone levels and improve sperm quality, making it more likely for them to father a child.

But hold your horses (or should I say, storks)—every journey to parenthood is unique, and results may vary. It's important to have an open and honest conversations with your fertility doctor about your specific situation and any potential fertility improvements.

Also remember, fertility is a team sport! Your partner's health and fertility also play a role in this grand baby-making symphony. So, it's a fantastic opportunity for both of you to join forces, embark on a healthier lifestyle together, and create a solid foundation for your future family.

Now, hold on tight and don't forget to take a peek at the section where we dive into the delightful topic of the best time to embark on your pregnancy journey post-sleeve. It's like finding the hidden treasure on your post-op map!

13. Does insurance cover sleeve gastrectomy?

Ah, insurance coverage—everyone's favorite topic! Brace yourselves for a few ups and downs as we take a look at the circus of insurance and sleeve gastrectomy.

So, here's the deal. Insurance coverage for sleeve gastrectomy is about as predictable as a squirrel on a unicycle. It varies from plan to plan, policy to policy. It's like playing a game of "Will They or Won't They?" with your insurance company.

Now, let's talk about those criteria. First up, we have the BMI requirement. Your BMI should be high enough to send a distress signal to the insurance gods. We're talking a BMI of 35 or maybe even 40, depending on your insurance plan. It's like having a flashing neon sign that says, "Hey, I've got some serious excess weight here!"

But that's not all, folks! You must prove that you've tried everything under the sun to shed those pounds. Think medically supervised diets, exercise programs, and all those other weight loss methods that make you question your life choices. It's like presenting a weight loss résumé to your insurance company, complete with references and testimonials.

Oh, and let's not forget the fun part—obesity-related health conditions. You need some legit medical issues to spice up the mix. Diabetes, high blood pressure, sleep apnea, and joint problems are all acts the insurance ringleader will look for when reviewing your case.

Now, hold on tight, because here comes the bariatric surgeon evaluation. It's like going through a series of obstacle courses to prove that sleeve gastrectomy is medically necessary. You'll be poked, prodded, and examined from every angle. It's like a doctor version of America's Got Talent, where they judge your eligibility for surgery. You might even need clearances from more than one doctor!

But wait, there's more! Before you dive headfirst into sleeve gastrectomy, you'll need to crack open that insurance policy and decode it like a secret message. Look for words like deductibles, co-pays, and out-of-pocket expenses. It's like deciphering a cryptic puzzle that only the insurance industry could create. Fun times, right? That's why many insurance companies have nurses and/or patient advocates on staff to help you answers those questions. Now, they may not advertise these experts, so you'll want to call and ask for them.

And just when you thought you were ready to roll, some insurance plans may require pre-authorization or prior approval. It's like getting permission to enter the sleeve gastrectomy club. So, you'll want to make sure you have all your paperwork in order because you don't want to be stuck outside the party, banging on the door.

Now I do not want you to stress yourself too much. When it comes to sleeve gastrectomy or any surgical procedure, most places have a helpful team to guide you through the whole process. They're like your support crew! From the moment you start considering the surgery, these awesome folks are there to answer your questions, explain what's gonna go down, and help you prepare for it all.

So, there you have it, folks! Insurance coverage for sleeve gastrectomy is a whirlwind adventure full of surprises, requirements, and a dash of frustration. But again, most surgical practices have got your back every step of the way!

14. How much does sleeve gastrectomy cost?

Worried about how much this surgery will cost? You're probably one of those budget-savvy folks! Let's dive into the wallet-walloping world of sleeve gastrectomy expenses. Now, if you're lucky enough to have insurance, make sure you do the insurance tango with them and your hospital to figure out that expected copay and any other expenses. The previous section covers that, so you can skip this part.

But hey, if you're one of those insurance-less daredevils out there, this part's for you!

Alright, brace yourselves, because the cost of sleeve gastrectomy is like a rollercoaster ride—lots of ups and downs. We're talking about location, healthcare facility, surgeon fees, and all those fancy pre-op tests. It's a seemingly uphill journey full of expenses! But hold on to your wallets because the price can vary like crazy. We're talking different prices in different countries and even within different regions.

Now, in the good old USA, you're looking at a price tag ranging from $10,000 to $20,000 or more. Yep, that's some serious cash. But hey, that figure includes everything from hospital fees to surgeon fees, anesthesia costs, pre-op tests, and even follow-up visits. Before you let out a sigh of relief though, let me tell you a secret: these numbers are just guesstimates. They can go up, down, with little warning.

But wait, there's hope for all you penny pinchers! If you don't have insurance or your insurance decides to ghost you on the surgery, many bariatric programs offer payment options. Yep, they know how to be a little flexible. So, don't fret, my frugal friends. There's always a way to finance that sleeve gastrectomy dream of yours. Just few options to suggest:

- Personal Loan: You can explore getting a personal loan from a bank or a reputable online lender. This way, you can borrow the amount needed for the surgery and repay it over time through fixed monthly installments.

- Credit Cards: If you have a credit card with a sufficient credit limit and reasonable interest rates, it could be used to cover the cost of the surgery. Just be cautious about carrying a balance and ensure you have a plan to pay it off promptly. Additionally, you might explore applying for a credit card that offers a 0% interest introductory period. This way, you can make use of the interest-free time to repay the card within that period, avoiding any interest charges altogether. It's a smart move if you can manage to pay it back on time!

- Care Credit Program: The Care Credit program is designed specifically for healthcare expenses. It acts like a credit card but is focused on medical services. It offers various financing options, including interest-free periods, making it a popular choice for covering medical procedures like sleeve gastrectomy.

Remember to review the terms and interest rates for each financing option carefully. It's essential to choose an option that aligns with your financial situation and allows you to manage the costs comfortably.

Alright, now let's talk about being a globetrotting medical tourist. I'll be upfront with you, folks. When it comes to your health, taking unnecessary risks isn't cool. Sleeve gastrectomy is a big deal – it's an investment in your well-being, and many people swear it's the best thing they ever did for themselves.

But let's be real – you don't want it to turn into a nightmare. Going for the cheapest option or hopping on a medical vacation might seem tempting, but it's not worth jeopardizing your health. Your well-being is top priority, no matter who you are!

Think about it like this – instead of splurging on a fancy car or an extravagant vacation, why not invest in yourself? Your health is priceless, and trust me, it's worth every penny.

So, don't rush into anything, do your research, and find a reputable, experienced team you can trust. Look for a place with a good track record, a supportive staff, and top-notch facilities. You all deserve the best when it comes to your health, and making the right choice now will pay off big time in the long run.

Now, who's ready to slim down their waistline without slimming down their bank account? Let's make this weight loss journey a financial success story, too!

15. How long does a sleeve gastrectomy surgery take?

Alright, let's break down the timeline of this sleeve gastrectomy shindig.

1-2 Hours of Surgery Bliss: The length of the actual surgery depends on a bunch of factors. It's tailored to each person's unique case and the surgeon's skills. On average, you'll be snoozing away for about 1 to 2 hours while the magic happens. The surgical team will make some small cuts in your belly, work their surgical wizardry, and reshape your stomach into a fancy sleeve-like shape. Think of it as a high-end makeover for your insides.

But Wait, There's More: The clock doesn't stop there. The surgery time only counts the bits happening in the operating room. Before and after the surgery, there are some necessary steps to take. You'll meet with the dietitian, get a medical assessment, and go through pre-operative tests. It's all part of the grand preparation to ensure you're physically ready and all safety precautions are in place. You must dot those Is and cross those Ts, my friend!

Under the Anesthesia Spell: During the surgery, you'll be knocked out cold under general anesthesia. No pain, no discomfort, just a nice nap while the surgeon does their thing.

Recovery Room Shenanigans: After the surgery, it's time for the recovery room party! You'll be whisked away to a special area where the medical staff will keep a watchful eye on you. This VIP lounge is where they make sure you wake up from anesthesia like a champ and that all your vital signs are stable. You'll hang out there for about 1 to 4 hours, soaking up that post-surgery care and attention.

Hospital Staycation: Don't pack your bags just yet! While the surgery itself may be a relatively short affair, the recovery is where the real action happens. You'll be a guest at the hospital for one to two days, receiving all the TLC you need to heal and get back on your feet. The doctors and nurses will be by your side, monitoring your progress, managing any pain, and guiding you through the early stages of recovery. They'll give you all the juicy deets on what to eat, how to take your meds, and what activities are a no-go.

Healing Time: Now, here's the kicker—recovery time can be like a box of chocolates. Each piece is a little different, and you might not know exactly what it's going to be. Some people may bounce back and feel ready to conquer the world after just a few days. They're like the speed demons of healing. But hey, others might need a few weeks to get back in the groove. It's important to follow your healthcare team's advice, attend those follow-up visits like a champ, and keep the lines of communication open. If you have worries or burning questions, don't be shy- let your team know.

So, there you have it, the timeline of sleeve gastrectomy from start to finish. Just remember, it's not just about the surgery itself; it's about the whole recovery journey. Take it easy, listen to your healthcare team, and before you know it, you'll be strutting your stuff as the fabulous, lighter version of yourself!

16. Can sleeve gastrectomy be performed as a minimally invasive procedure?

Picture this: Instead of a big old slash on your abdomen, sleeve gastrectomy takes a more subtle approach. It's like a covert mission with laparoscopic or robotic techniques. The surgeon will make a few small incisions, like secret entrances for his instruments to sneak in. It's like performing surgery with a spy team!

But wait, there's more! The surgical team invites a special guest—a thin camera—to guide the surgeon through the operation. It's like having a high-tech tour guide showing the way. And with the help of those nifty surgical instruments, the surgeon works their magic, removing a portion of your stomach to create a smaller, sleeve-shaped tummy. It's like a stomach remodeling show, transforming it into a sleek, slimmed-down version!

Now, let's talk perks. These minimally invasive techniques come with a bunch of advantages. First, the incisions are like tiny battle scars, hardly noticeable. So, sad to say you won't be rocking a massive surgical scar you can use as a conversation starter. But, you'll experience less post-operative pain, which means you can ditch those painkillers faster than you can say "recovery mode activated."

And here's the real kicker—shorter hospital stays and faster recovery times. It's like getting an express ticket out of the hospital and back to your regular life. Who needs to be stuck in a hospital bed when you can be out there, conquering the world with your newfound sleeve-shaped stomach?

Oh, and let's not forget about the bonus points. Minimally invasive procedures generally have a lower risk of complications and infections. It's like having a protective shield against the sneaky dangers lurking in the surgical world. Safety first, my friends!

Now, here's a little tip: when you're looking for a surgeon. Make sure they're all about that minimally invasive life. Although open sleeve gastrectomies—the ones with the massive incision—are like a VHS tape in a world of streaming services, there might be few surgeons who still offer this method. You'll want to avoid those and embrace the wonders of laparoscopic or robotic surgery, my friends!

So, there you have it, folks! Sleeve gastrectomy takes a leap into the world of minimally invasive surgery, making it a sleek, scar-free, and speedy journey. It's like upgrading from clunky old technology to a sleek, high-tech version. Get ready to rock that sleeve-shaped stomach and conquer the world, one small incision at a time!

17. I have a band. Can I have a sleeve gastrectomy?

The Gastric Band weight loss surgery, also known as adjustable gastric band, involves placing an adjustable silicone band around the upper part of the stomach. It creates a smaller upper pouch, restricting food intake and promoting weight loss. The band can be adjusted over time, and the procedure is reversible. However, it typically leads to slower and more gradual weight loss compared to other bariatric surgeries.

Overall, you won't catch me endorsing those adjustable bands! I've seen so many of them come back to haunt patients after being put in by other surgeons. It's not uncommon for folks with these bands to experience heartburn and have trouble swallowing. And to top it off, there's a real risk of gaining back the weight you worked so hard to lose. So, my friendly advice is to steer clear of the bands – nope, not on my watch! I don't even offer them as an option to my patients because I believe in the power of the other bariatric surgeries! Back to the sleeve for example, it's like a hormone powerhouse compared to the band! It causes a more significant change in your hormones, resulting in more weight loss and less chance of gaining that weight back!

So, if you've already got a band and you're wondering if you can switch it up with a sleeve gastrectomy? Here's the deal: Yes, it's possible to have a sleeve gastrectomy even if you've got a band hanging around in your tummy. It's like saying, "Adios, band! I'm upgrading to a sleek and slender sleeve!"

But hold on tight because there are a few things to consider. Converting your band to a sleeve gastrectomy is a popular option. The procedure involves removing the band and transforming your stomach into a sleeve-shaped wonder. It's like going from a band that restrains your eating habits to a sleeve that helps you conquer those calories head-on thru restriction AND hormonal changes!

But here's the fun part: If you're thinking of converting your band, some surgeons (including me) prefer a conversion to gastric bypass instead of a sleeve gastrectomy, if you are a good candidate. The gastric bypass (more about it later) will help you 1- eat less, 2- change your hormones 3- help you absorb fewer calories (something the sleeve does not do)!

Now, keep in mind that every conversion is a unique journey. Those revisional surgeries tend to be more complex and carry more risks compared to undergoing a straightforward sleeve or bypass. It's important to have a good chat with your surgeon about the best approach for you. They'll be the expert who guides you through this band-to-sleeve transformation process. They'll help you weigh the pros and cons, answer all your burning questions, and set you up for success on your weight loss adventure.

18. What does the pre-operative workup entail?

Alright, folks, grab a seat and prepare yourselves for the pre-op extravaganza! We've got a checklist longer than a giraffe's neck, but don't worry, I'll make it fun!

First up, we've got the initial consultation with your bariatric surgeon. They'll give you the lowdown on the surgery, the risks, the benefits, and answer all your burning questions. And be warned, they'll also give your medical history a thorough review, so be ready to spill the beans on any previous surgeries, chronic conditions, or allergies. Be ready to reveal all of your medical secrets! During the visit you'll receive all the juicy details about the surgical procedure, the expected outcomes, and potential risks and complications. Also we've got some lifestyle counseling coming your way. Get ready for the ultimate crash course in dietary changes, physical activity, and behavior modification. It's like a crash course in becoming a weight loss superstar!

Next, we're diving into the world of nutrition with a registered dietitian. They'll assess your current eating habits, nutritional status, and figure out any special dietary needs you may have. It's like a culinary detective trying to crack the case of your diet.

Now, let's not forget about the psychological evaluation. We need to make sure you're mentally prepared for this wild ride. A mental health professional will assess your readiness for the surgery, make sure you understand the lifestyle changes ahead, and provide some much-needed support. It's like getting a mental health check-up before the big weight loss party!

Now, get ready for the vampire brigade because blood tests are next! They'll check your red and white blood cell counts, hemoglobin levels, platelet count, and more. It's like a blood runway show where your cells get to strut their stuff.

Also, time to take a peek at your heart with an electrocardiogram (ECG). They'll record the electrical activity of your heart, making sure everything's ticking along just right.

Now, get ready for some imaging studies. Chest X-rays and echocardiograms may be on the agenda, giving your organs a chance to shine under the spotlight.

And don't forget the star of the show—the abdominal ultrasound! It's time to assess that gallbladder for any unwanted visitors like gallstones. If you do have those, your surgeon might discuss removing the gallbladder during your sleeve surgery to prevent possible future complications from the stones.

Now, prepare for an endoscopic adventure! A flexible tube with a camera will journey through your throat and into your stomach, giving a close-up view of any abnormalities. It's like an exploratory mission through your own personal cave of wonders. More about endoscopy later.

And last, but not least, we have sleep studies. If you have snoring or sleep apnea symptoms, get ready to have your sleep quality analyzed.

Phew! That was quite the pre-op extravaganza, my friends. But hey, by going through this long checklist, you're setting yourself up for a safe and successful sleeve gastrectomy. So, let's get those boxes checked and embrace the journey to a healthier, happier you!

You can get a copy of my own preoperative check list on my website DoctorKudsi.com

19. Will I need to quit smoking before sleeve gastrectomy?

Ah, the sizzling question of whether you should bid farewell to the smoky puffs before your sleeve gastrectomy.

Now, let's clear the smoke and set the stage: Smoking and surgery don't exactly go hand-in-hand like a dance duo. In other words, not the best combo!

Smoking can increase the risk of complications during and after surgery. It's like inviting the party crasher of healing delays and potential lung issues to your recovery bash. So, consider this your opportunity to kick that smoking habit to the curb and show it who's boss!

Quitting is easier said than done, and we all know that. It's like wrestling with a stubborn kangaroo while attempting a graceful ballet routine. So, don't hesitate to seek support from healthcare professionals, nicotine replacement therapies, or even a support group of ex-smokers. Sometimes, we need all the help we can get!

But hey, here's a secret tip: Channel that "quitting smoking" energy into something positive and enjoyable. Find a new hobby, learn a musical instrument, or dive into a new adventure that tickles your fancy. You'll be amazed at how awesome it feels to redirect that energy toward something that brings you joy and satisfaction.

So, while quitting smoking before your sleeve gastrectomy may be challenging, it's a move that will set you up for a healthier, smoother, and more successful surgery and recovery. Embrace the journey, arm yourself with support and humor, and kick that smoking habit to the curb like a true champion!

20. Why do I need pre-operative upper endoscopy before sleeve gastrectomy?

So, before we go all "slicing and dicing" with the sleeve gastrectomy, let me tell you why I'm a big fan of pre-operative upper endoscopy. First off, it's like giving your stomach a little fashion show—checking out its lining, making sure it's all healthy and fabulous. No ulcers or polyps allowed, darlings! We want a safe and successful sleeve gastrectomy, after all.

Now, here's where things get interesting. Ever heard of a hiatal hernia? It's like your stomach playing a little game of peek-a-boo through your diaphragm into your chest. Not a good look, right? Endoscopy can help us spot that hernia and plan to repair it during the sleeve gastrectomy. But hey, if it's a real big hernia causing trouble like problem swallowing or heartburn, we might have to switch to the "gastric bypass" instead— as it has less chance of a recurrence of the hernia and less chance of causing heartburn in the future, guaranteed! More about gastric bypass later!

And wait, there's more! We're not just window shopping, we're going full-on detective mode. Biopsies, my friends! We're talking tissue samples from suspicious areas. We don't want any surprises down the road, so let's make sure we rule out any pre-cancerous or cancerous conditions. This is particularly important for if you have heartburn or are greater risk of gastric cancer. Safety first, people!

So, remember, before you jump into the sleeve gastrectomy whirlwind, let's give your tummy the ultimate VIP treatment. It's all about being in tip-top shape before we start this health improvement journey.

It's important to mention that not all surgeons will deem upper endoscopy necessary prior to your surgery. However, for my patients, I consider it a crucial step and require it as part of the preparation process.

21. Why do I need to undergo a psychological evaluation before sleeve gastrectomy?

So, sleeve gastrectomy is definitely a big decision, big changes, and yeah, even a little post-op stress. But fear not, because before you take that plunge, we've got a psychological evaluation in store for you. It may sound scary, but there are very good reasons for examining your mental well-being.

First off, we want to make sure you're mentally fit for this weight loss adventure. We're checking for any emotional hurdles like depression, anxiety, or any undiagnosed eating disorder. It's all about setting you up for success and making sure you're ready to handle the ups and downs that come with the post-operative lifestyle changes.

But hey, it's not all negative business! We also want to know what's motivating you. We'll chat about realistic goals, potential challenges, and the fact that this isn't just a quick fix. It's a lifelong commitment, my friend.

Now, let's talk coping strategies. Weight loss surgery means shaking things up, especially in the food department. We want to know how you handle stress, emotions, and those pesky cravings. And don't worry, we're not just here to point out your weak spots. We'll help you develop some killer strategies to navigate the twists and turns of this weight loss journey. Stress ball? Check. Ice cream emergency hotline? Double check.

But wait, there's more! The evaluation also comes with support and counseling. Got concerns, fears, or emotional baggage related to the surgery? Your team will guide you, educate you, and provide resources to tackle the emotional roller coaster that comes with shedding those pounds. You won't be alone in this, I promise.

Last, but not least, we must identify any risk factors. We want to make sure you've got a solid support system in place and that you're not the kind of person who throws medical recommendations out the window. And hey, if you need a little extra mental health support during your post-op journey, we've got your back. No judgment, just lots of help to keep you on track.

So, there you have it! The psychological evaluation is all about getting your mind in the game, preparing you for the challenges ahead, and keeping your mental and emotional well-being in check. So, get ready to face those lifestyle changes head-on and remember, you're never alone on this wild weight loss ride!

22. Can sleeve gastrectomy be combined with other weight loss procedures?

Oh, we're getting fancy with our weight loss procedures now! So, let's talk about combining sleeve gastrectomy with other procedures and discuss revisional surgery. It's like a tag team match for your weight loss goals!

First up, we've got the duodenal switch (DS). It's like a sleeve gastrectomy with a twist—literally! We modify your intestines to make weight loss even more hardcore. It's like taking your stomach size down a notch and rerouting your intestines to play hard to get with calories and nutrients. This will definitely decrease the absorption of calories and nutrients. Talk about a double whammy!

Next in the ring, we've got the gastric bypass! This approach involves two stages and is designed for individuals aiming to achieve a greater degree of weight loss than what could be accomplished through either sleeve gastrectomy or bypass surgery alone. First, you start with the sleeve gastrectomy, shrinking that stomach down like it's on a crash diet. And then, at a later date, after you've achieved the maximum weight loss that the sleeve would offer, you proceed with a gastric bypass. This dynamic duo is usually reserved for those with seriously high body mass index (BMI) or those with some complicated medical conditions. You must earn your way to this combo!

But wait, there's more! We've got revisional surgeries in the mix, too. Picture this: You've had a previous weight loss procedure like an adjustable gastric band, but things aren't going quite according to plan with heartburn, difficulty swallowing, and/or not losing enough weight. Well, it's time for the sleeve gastrectomy to come to the rescue! The band can be removed, and a sleeve is done. Now discuss with your surgeon as some surgeons prefer converting the band to a bypass.

Now, here's a little secret for you. Combining procedures and revisional surgeries might sound like a piece of cake, but it's important to know that those come with some extra risks and complications. It's like adding a few more obstacles to your weight loss journey. So, make sure you're fully informed and you and your surgeon agree the rewards are greater than the risks!

So, there you have it, folks! Sleeve gastrectomy is no longer flying solo. It can team up with other weight loss procedures like a true weight loss superhero. Just remember, it's all about finding the right combo for you, considering your unique circumstances and goals. Get ready to knock out those pounds and show 'em who's the heavyweight champion of weight loss!

23. Can weight loss medications be used instead of sleeve gastrectomy?

At this point, you might be thinking you'd rather try some pills than a full-on surgery. We're about to have a showdown between weight loss medications and sleeve gastrectomy. Let's get ready to rumble!

In this corner, we have weight loss medications, the little pills that promise to help you shed those pounds. They're like the sidekicks in your weight loss journey, doing their best to reduce your appetite, make you feel full, or mess with how your body absorbs nutrients. But here's the catch—they're like the backup dancers, good for some moves, but they cannot be the stars of the show.

These weight loss medications are usually prescribed to folks with a BMI around 27 to 30, or even higher. They're like the extra push you need when the scale is stuck and you're feeling a bit meh. But let's be real here, they don't lead to as much weight loss as sleeve gastrectomy. It's like adding on a touch of lip gloss compared to a full-on stomach makeover.

Now, let's talk about the weight loss medication crew. They're not for everyone and can have some funky side effects. And guess what? Once you stop taking them, the weight might just waltz right back into your life, uninvited. Talk about a rude guest!

And in the other corner, we have the heavyweight champion, sleeve gastrectomy! This surgery is like the ultimate transformation, making your stomach smaller so you feel full with less food. Plus, it's a more permanent solution that helps you lose a lot of weight and keep it off. Take that, weight loss medications!

But hold up, folks! We don't need to throw weight loss medications out of the ring completely. They can still be a valuable sidekick to sleeve gastrectomy, like the extra sprinkle on top of a delicious cake. No matter if you go for the sleeve gastrectomy or not, you'll always have the backup option to use weight loss meds if you need 'em.

So there you have it, folks! Weight loss medications and sleeve gastrectomy battling it out in the ring. While weight loss medications do their best to assist, sleeve gastrectomy takes the crown for long-lasting and effective weight loss. Choose wisely, my friends, and may the pounds be shed ever in your favor!

24. Is sleeve gastrectomy reversible?

Alright, let's dive into the wild world of sleeve gastrectomy revisions and conversions. We discussed some of those earlier but let's dig deeper! You see, this weight loss journey can sometimes take unexpected turns, and that's where these funky revision surgeries come into play.

When Things Go Wonky: Normally, sleeve gastrectomy is a forever kind of deal. It permanently shrinks the size and shape of your stomach, so there's no going back. But hey, life happens, and there are rare situations where a revision or conversion surgery might be on the table. It's like a special menu item you never thought you'd need to order.

Complications, Anyone?: Sometimes, our bodies have a mind of their own and decide to throw a tantrum after sleeve gastrectomy. You might experience complications or side effects that seriously mess with your health or quality of life. Think intense acid reflux, persistent vomiting, or a stricture (narrow sleeve) that just won't cooperate. If these issues persist despite trying other treatments (like endoscopic interventions), your surgeon might consider a revisional surgery. It's like hitting the reset button, but with a fancy name—Roux En Y gastric bypass is the most common conversion option. It's like giving your stomach a makeover 2.0. More about gastric bypass next!

Weight Loss Woes: Now, let's talk about those times when the scale isn't playing nice. Sleeve gastrectomy is usually a pretty effective weight loss solution, but hey, there are those rare instances where the pounds just won't budge or decide to come back for a reunion tour. If you've given it your all, danced with lifestyle changes, and tried other interventions, but weight loss still eludes you, a revisional surgery might be on the horizon. Picture a weight loss remix—converting to duodenal switch or revisiting our friend, gastric bypass. It's like shaking things up to find that sweet spot.

Remember, these revision and conversion surgeries are not your everyday occurrences. They're like the unicorns of sleeve gastrectomy, appearing only in special circumstances. Your surgeon will carefully evaluate your situation and consider all the factors before busting out the revision playbook.

So, embrace the quirks of the weight loss journey, and if you find yourself in the land of revisions and conversions, know that there are options out there to keep the adventure going. Just make sure to have a chat with your surgeon and rock that revised path with confidence!

25. What is Roux En Y gastric bypass?

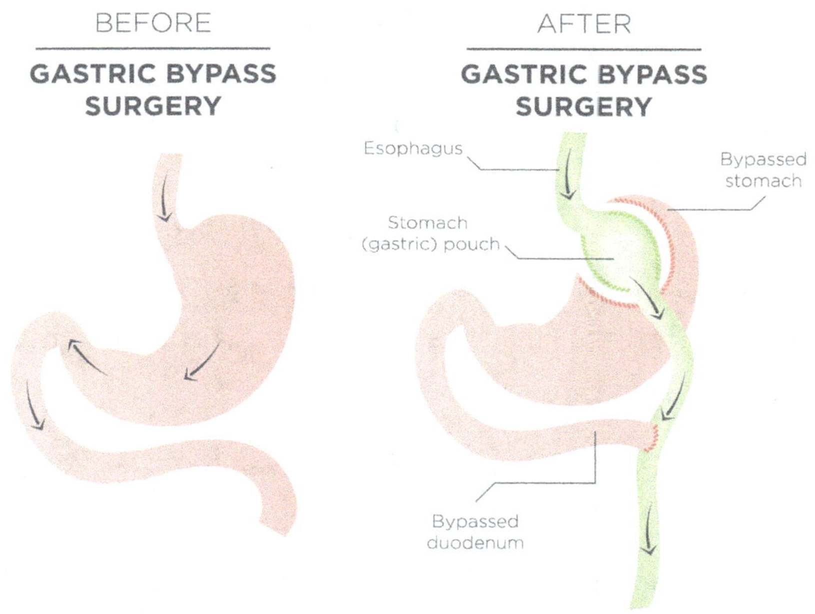

Dividing and Conquering: So, picture this: We surgeons transform the stomach into a cool two-section wonderland during gastric bypass. We whip out our surgical magic and create a smaller stomach gastric upper pouch, while the lower section stays large and in charge called the bypassed stomach. Then, we get creative and connect a part of the small intestine to the upper pouch, creating a shiny new bypass lane for food to take. Talk about a culinary detour!

Size Matters: Now, here's the fun part—this smaller upper pouch has some strict rules. It can only handle a tiny amount of food at a time, meaning you'll be singing a different tune when it comes to portion sizes. Say goodbye to massive meals and hello to bite-sized portions. It's like having a stomach that says, "I'll take a little sip of that, thank you very much." With less food in the mix, those pesky calories take a backseat, and weight loss becomes the star of the show.

Nutrient Ninja: But wait, there's more! The bypassed section of the intestine becomes the superhero of the story. The food that you eat will not pass thru the bypassed stomach and part of the intestines reducing the absorption of nutrients and calories from the food you eat. It's like having a secret agent inside your body, sneakily swiping away some of those calories, making them disappear into thin air. It's like magic, but with a surgical twist. So, even if you indulge in a delicious meal, your body won't absorb as many calories as it used to. Talk about a weight loss double whammy!

Gastric Bypass vs. Sleeve Gastrectomy: Time for a battle of the weight loss giants! Gastric bypass usually takes the crown when it comes to greater weight loss. It's like the heavyweight champion of the surgical weight loss world. And hey, if you're dealing with acid reflux after sleeve gastrectomy, gastric bypass swoops in like a superhero to save the day. It's like having a gastric knight in shining armor, putting that pesky acid reflux in its place.

But Hold On: While gastric bypass is a weight loss superstar, it's important to mention that it can be a bit trickier and comes with more potential long-term complications compared to sleeve gastrectomy. Some of the possible long-term complications include nutrients deficiency (since you are not absorbing some of the nutrients that you are eating), the possibility of bowel blockage or having an ulcer where we connect the intestines to the upper stomach pouch.

So, there you have it, the wild and whimsical world of gastric bypass. It's a surgical journey filled with divided stomachs, bypassed intestines, and a whole lot of weight loss magic. Just remember, consult with your surgeon to determine if this adventure is the right fit for you. Happy bypassing!

26. What is a Duodenal Switch?

Hold onto your funny bones, folks, because we're about to dive into the zany world of duodenal switch! Get ready for a wild ride of stomach size reduction, intestinal rerouting, and weight loss wonders.

There are two main types for duodenal switch: the traditional, or "biliopancreatic diversion with duodenal switch" (BPD/DS), and the "single-anastomosis duodenal switch" (SADI-S).

The traditional duodenal switch (BPD/DS) is like a two-part deal.

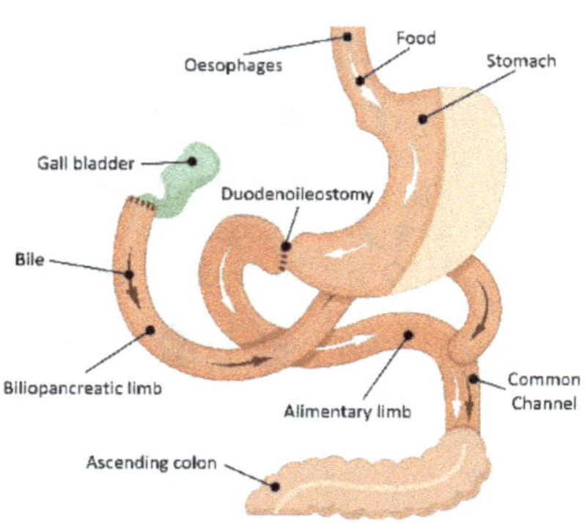

The first part is similar to a sleeve gastrectomy where part of the stomach is removed to make it smaller.

The second part is where we reroute your small intestine to change how your body absorbs food, meaning you absorb fewer calories and nutrients.

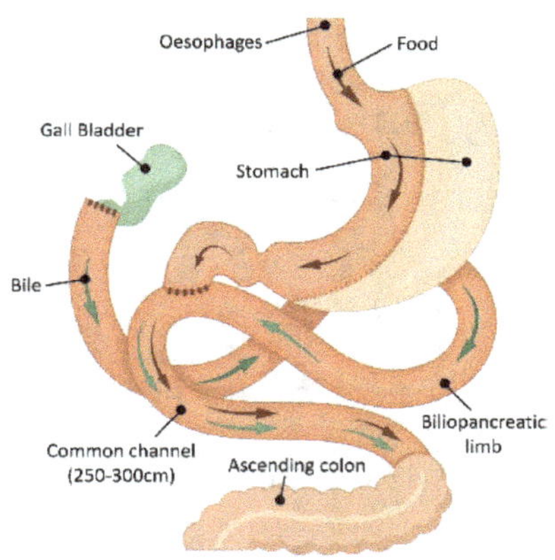

The single-anastomosis duodenal switch (SADI-S), on the other hand, is a simpler version.

It's a little bit like the traditional one, but instead of making two new connections (anastomoses) in your intestines, we only make one.

This version is a bit newer and is usually easier on the patient with less surgical risk.

So now let's discuss Sleeve-to-Duodenal Switch Conversion: So, let's say you already had a sleeve gastrectomy and now you're ready to take it to the next level. Fear not, my friend, because the conversion to duodenal switch is here to save the day. Since your stomach size is already reduced, the surgery becomes a bit like a VIP rerouting party for your intestines. We'll just focus on limiting caloric absorption and giving your weight loss journey an extra boost. It's like taking a detour from the detour. Clever, right?

Now more about acid Reflux and conversion to Gastric Bypass: just like we mentioned earlier, if you're dealing with side effects from the sleeve, like acid reflux, then it's time for the gastric bypass. With gastric bypass we create a smaller stomach pouch. This new, tiny stomach has less acid in it. Less acid means less chance for it to flow back up to your esophagus (the tube that connects your mouth to your stomach). Hence less acid reflux.

The Complexity Conundrum: Now, let's not forget, the duodenal switch is the most intricate dance routine of weight loss surgeries. It's a bit more complex than your average sleeve gastrectomy. And yes, with complexity comes the possibility of long-term complications. But hey, with the right surgeon and your own research, you'll navigate those complexities like a pro!

So, there you have it, the wonderfully wacky world of duodenal switch. It's a combination of stomach size reduction, intestinal rerouting, and weight loss enchantment. Just remember, consult with your surgeon and know what's best for you—it's the secret ingredient for a successful journey. Happy switching!

27. What are the potential risks and complications of sleeve gastrectomy?

Let's dive into the world of sleeve gastrectomy complications. It can seem like a rollercoaster ride with some twists and turns. But let's explore these risks.

First off, let's discuss the general risks that come with any surgery. You've got your classic bleeding, infection, and adverse reactions to anesthesia. Oh, and let's not forget the possibility of blood clots or accidentally injuring some nearby organs. When you think about all these risks, it might seem like a high-stakes game of surgical roulette, but don't worry—the odds are in your favor!

Now, let's talk about leaks. No, not the juicy celebrity gossip kind, but the small risk of leakage from the staple line where the surgeon divides the stomach. Just imagine it like a garden hose with a tiny hole, leaking water. Now, this is rare, but it's serious when it does happen. You might feel some pain, feel sick or even run a fever. Usually fixing leaks will require some intervention like endoscopies or drain placement.

Oh, and here's a fun one—strictures! A stricture is a narrow passage in the middle of your sleeve which will usually cause difficulty swallowing food. Another rare event which might require a few endoscopies for dilation or, in rare cases, even another surgery.

Next up, we have the notorious acid reflux. Some "lucky" individuals might experience an increase in acid reflux or heartburn after the surgery. But fear not, these symptoms are usually manageable with medication, dietary changes, or some intentional lifestyle modifications. And hey, worst-case scenario, you might even score an invite to the gastric bypass conversion crowd!

Now, onto nutritional deficiencies. Your body might decide to throw a curveball and make you miss out on some important vitamins and minerals like B12, iron, and calcium. But fear not, regular monitoring and the use of fancy supplements will keep you on track.

You may have heard about the thrilling world of dumping syndrome! It's like a secret club that's more common after gastric bypass but occasionally welcomes sleeve patients, too. It's when your food decides to sprint from your stomach to your small intestine like an overexcited marathon runner. Cue the nausea, sweating, weakness, dizziness, and the grand finale—a diarrhea extravaganza. But fear not, you can manage this by eating smaller, more frequent meals and avoiding those pesky trigger foods.

Oh, and let's not forget the gallstones. Rapid weight loss might turn you into a rock collector, but not the cool kind. Nope, we're talking gallstones, my friend. And if things get rocky, you might even score a bonus round of gallbladder removal during your sleeve adventure. Again, some surgeons will offer you gallbladder removal during sleeve gastrectomy if you already have stones in your gallbladder.

Last, but not least, there's weight regain. It's like that annoying friend who crashes your weight loss party uninvited. But don't worry, with the power of dietary and lifestyle changes, you can kick them out and keep the weight off. It's all about maintenance, my friend! Also, as previously discussed you can always go on weight loss medication to help lose the unwanted weight.

So, there you have it—sleeve gastrectomy complications. Just remember, the risks are relatively low compared to the amazing benefits that await you on this weight-loss journey.

28. What are the potential risks of anesthesia during sleeve gastrectomy?

Ah, anesthesia, the magical potion that sends you off to dreamland during sleeve gastrectomy! But like any spell, it comes with a few risks. Don't worry, though, I'll break it down for you!

First up, we have the usual suspects: allergic reactions. Just like some people are allergic to bees or cotton candy (weird, right?), there's a small chance you could have an allergic reaction to the anesthesia drugs. But fear not; the anesthesiologists are always prepared for such situations. They'll monitor you closely and have the antidotes ready. They're ready to save the day like superheroes in scrubs!

Next on our list is the drowsy aftermath. Anesthesia can leave you feeling as groggy as a bear in hibernation. You might experience some lingering dizziness, confusion, or even nausea when you wake up. But fear not; these side effects are usually temporary and fade away!

Anesthesia can also occasionally cause complications during or after surgery such as breathing difficulties, changes in blood pressure, or even heart issues. But don't panic! These risks are rare, and the medical team is there to juggle any potential problems with their expert skills.

29. How long will I need to stay in the hospital after sleeve gastrectomy?

Ah, the million-dollar question! How long are you going to rock that hospital gown after your sleeve gastrectomy?

Typically, after a sleeve gastrectomy, the average hospital stay is around one to three nights. Think about like a mini vacation where you don't have to worry about cooking or doing the dishes! You'll have a team of healthcare superheroes checking on you, making sure you're recovering like a champ.

The length of your stay can vary depending on several factors. If you're bouncing back like a rubber ball and your surgeon is impressed with your progress, you might be out of there faster than you can say "sleeve gastrectomy superstar!" On the flip side, if your body needs a little more time to recover or if any unexpected complications arise, you might be extending your hospital stay like a VIP guest demanding extra room service. Hey, who doesn't love a few extra hospital Jell-C cups, right?

During your hospital stay, you'll have plenty of time to relax, catch up on your favorite TV shows, and become best friends with the hospital staff. They'll be there to guide you through the early stages of your recovery, making sure you're getting the right pain medications, keeping an eye on your incisions, and making sure you're up and moving like a groove master.

And hey, don't forget about the post-op diet adventure that awaits you! While you're in the hospital, you'll start with sips of clear liquids, like a classy connoisseur of broth and Jell-O. Gradually, you'll level up to thicker liquids. It's like going from liquid gold to smooth food heaven! Your healthcare team will be there, cheering you on and giving you all the tips and tricks for navigating this culinary journey.

So, get ready for a hospital stay that's shorter than binge-watching your favorite show but long enough to give you a taste of that hospital life. Embrace the attention, rock that gown with style, and get ready to embark on the next chapter of your sleeve gastrectomy adventure.

30. How long is the recovery period after sleeve gastrectomy?

Alright, folks, let's talk about the recovery period after sleeve gastrectomy! It's like a journey to bounce back and embrace your new stomach situation. So, get ready to recover in style!

First things first, the hospital stay. It's like a mini vacation, except you're trading sandy beaches for a comfy hospital bed. Depending on your situation and your surgeon's recommendation, you'll be chilling in the hospital for 1 to 3 days. Don't forget to bring your finest pajamas and make the most of the room service!

Now, let's talk about physical activity. It's like a slow-motion workout video, starting with short walks that make snails look speedy. You'll gradually level up to more moderate exercises, feeling like a superhero conquering the world, one step at a time. Just remember, you're not training for the Olympics (unless you are, then go for gold!), so take it easy and let your body heal. You can find my post bariatric surgery exercise program on my website DoctorKudsi.com

Ah, pain and discomfort—the not-so-glamorous side of recovery. Pain is a pesky little reminder that your body just went through some serious changes. But fear not, your surgeon will provide you with pain management strategies. Think of it as a survival kit filled with magical potions to keep discomfort at bay. And remember, pain is temporary, but the fabulous results are forever!

Let's not forget the dietary changes. It might seem like learning to eat like you did as a baby, starting with a clear liquid diet and slowly adding more exciting consistencies to your plate. From sipping broths like a fancy connoisseur to conquering pureed foods like a master chef, you'll rock this new gastronomic adventure. Embrace the creativity in the kitchen and make those purees look like culinary masterpieces! You can find some meal plan ideas on my website DoctorKudsi.com

Regular follow-up appointments are a must during the recovery period. Think of these visits as recurring dates with your healthcare team, where they monitor your progress, address any concerns or complications, and provide guidance.

Returning to work is the moment when you rejoin the real world. It's like leaving your cozy recovery bubble and stepping back into the daily grind. Some lucky individuals can get back to work within 1 to 2 weeks if their job involves more brainpower than heavy lifting. But if your job requires Hulk-like strength, you might need a bit more recovery time. Embrace the extra vacation days, my friend!

Remember, recovery from sleeve gastrectomy is like a dance—sometimes slow, sometimes challenging, but always worth it. Patience and commitment are your partners on this journey.

31. Will I need to have follow-up appointments after sleeve gastrectomy?

Hey there, follow-up superstar! You've got your very own fan club waiting to see you after your sleeve surgery. Those follow-up appointments are like the red-carpet events of your weight loss journey. Let's dive into the world of post-operative follow-ups, where you're the VIP:

First up, we have the initial post-operative visits. It's like a series of grand openings where your surgeon checks on your healing, tackles any complications, and makes sure you're adjusting like a pro to your new dietary and lifestyle changes.

But the fun doesn't stop there, my friend! You'll have regular check-ups with your bariatric surgeon and their marvelous multidisciplinary team. It's like having a squad of experts cheering you on and making sure you're rocking that weight loss journey. They'll see you more times than you can count, appearing like a Kardashian on a reality show marathon.

Oh, and get ready for some nutritional assessment action! They'll monitor your vitamin and mineral levels like a hawk and give you the lowdown on the right supplements to keep you glowing with health. You'll even get to meet a registered dietitian, like having your very own food guru guiding you through the culinary maze.

Also, your surgeon will be tracking your weight loss progress and making adjustments if needed. If the pounds are slow to say their goodbyes, they might even prescribe some weight loss medications. It's like having a secret weapon in your back pocket, ready to kick those stubborn pounds to the curb.

And let's not forget the behavioral support. Your surgeon knows that weight loss isn't just about the physical stuff —it's a mental and emotional journey, too. That's why they'll hook you up with counseling or support groups to address any emotional or psychological challenges if needed. They want to make sure your entourage has all the right people.

So, my friend, don't miss those follow-up appointments. Get ready to strut your stuff and show off your amazing progress.

32. How soon can I return to work after sleeve gastrectomy?

Now on to the eternal dilemma of returning to work after a sleeve gastrectomy! Let's dive into the nitty-gritty, shall we?

So, the norm is to feel tired for 2 to 6 weeks. That said, if you have an office job where you spend most of your time sitting at a desk, you might be able to bounce back to work as soon as 3 days! I am ok with my patients going back to work whenever they feel like it. After all, you won't be running marathons or lugging heavy equipment around. However, don't underestimate the power of those sneaky office snacks and tempting lunchroom treats. Keep your guard up, my friend! Remember, your new sleeve means you'll be eating smaller portions, so choose wisely and savor every bite.

Now back at it! Stay hydrated by keeping a water bottle at your desk, ready to conquer any thirst that dares to challenge you. As I mentioned previously, your main full-time job after surgery is drinking! Anything else comes next to it. You won't be able to do anything else if you end up being dehydrated and get admitted back to the hospital.

Now, if your job involves being out and about, like a construction worker or a tour guide, things might be a tad different. Your body will need some extra time to recover because physical labor can be demanding, and you don't want to strain those healing muscles, which could cause a hernia. Plus, being outdoors can also affect your hydration game. Sweating under the scorching sun or battling the elements might require some extra H2O intake. So, if your job is physically demanding or involves you being in extreme heat, you'll likely need a little more time off.

Whether you're rocking an office job or conquering the great outdoors, always listen to your body. It'll give you the cues you need to determine if you're ready to return to work. And don't forget to give yourself a pat on the back for undergoing such a transformative journey. The world is eagerly awaiting your triumphant return to the workforce, armed with your newfound health and slimming success! But, you don't want to make your grand entrance too soon!

33. How long do the effects of sleeve gastrectomy last?

Now, let's talk about longevity! The effects of sleeve gastrectomy can be like a loyal friend—they stick around for the long haul. Sleeve gastrectomy is considered a long-term solution for weight loss, and it can lead to significant and lasting weight reduction. Most people lose 50-70% of their excess weight within the first one to two years after surgery. The weight loss tends to stabilize after two to three years, but maintaining this weight loss requires consistent commitment to a healthy lifestyle, including good nutrition and regular exercise. You see, the magic of this procedure is that it jumpstarts your weight loss journey, but it's up to you to maintain it.

By adopting healthy eating habits, staying active, and working closely with your healthcare team, you can maximize the long-term benefits of sleeve gastrectomy.

Now, you might be wondering, "How long is this ride?" Well, my friend, the effects of sleeve gastrectomy can last a lifetime if you stick to your healthy lifestyle.

34. Will I experience any changes in appetite after sleeve gastrectomy?

Now, let's address the big question: Will you experience changes in appetite after the surgery? The short answer is... drumroll, please... YES, absolutely!

Picture this: You've got a stomach that's been transformed into a slender sleeve. It's like going from a big old buffet plate to a tiny appetizer dish. Your stomach size is reduced, which means it can't hold as much food as before. So, naturally, your appetite might take a nosedive. It's like your tummy saying, "Hey, we've got limited space here, buddy. You better be choosy about what you eat!"

But hold on because it's not just about the physical changes. As mentioned earlier, there's a little hormone called ghrelin that plays a sneaky role in all this. Ghrelin is like the ravenous gremlin that hangs out in your stomach, signaling your brain when you're hungry. After a sleeve gastrectomy, ghrelin levels tend to take a dip. It's like putting that gremlin on a strict diet! So, you might find yourself feeling less hungry and craving food less often. It's like your tummy and brain are finally on the same page, saying, "Hey, let's take it easy on the snacking, shall we?"

But wait, it's not always a smoother transition! While many people experience a decrease in appetite, it's not a guarantee. Some folks might still have moments of cravings and hunger. So, don't be surprised if your appetite decides to throw a curveball at you from time to time. It's all part of the journey of post-surgery eating!

Now, here's the important thing: Even though your appetite might change, it's crucial to maintain a healthy, balanced diet. It's like giving your body the fuel it needs without going overboard. Embrace those nutritious foods, enjoy the flavors, and listen to your body's signals.

35. Can sleeve gastrectomy affect my ability to absorb medications?

So, sleeve gastrectomy might have a few tricks up its sleeve, but it's unlikely to completely sabotage your medication absorption. Let's break it down, shall we?

When you undergo sleeve gastrectomy, your stomach becomes smaller. But don't worry, it doesn't vanish completely!

Now, medication absorption primarily takes place in the small intestine, not in the stomach. So even though your stomach has undergone a resizing act, the main stage for medication absorption remains intact and ready to perform its duties.

However, there's a small catch—a funny twist, if you will. Some medications are designed to be released and absorbed slowly in the stomach. With a smaller stomach, the speed at which these medications enter the small intestine might be altered. It's like trying to juggle water balloons while riding a unicycle—a bit tricky, but not impossible!

But don't panic just yet! Your doctors will take into account the changes in your anatomy and adjust your medications accordingly. They might opt for different formulations or dosages that ensure proper absorption.

So, while sleeve gastrectomy might add a sprinkle of unpredictability to your medication absorption, it's nothing a skilled medical team can't handle.

36. Are there any long-term complications associated with sleeve gastrectomy?

Sleeve gastrectomy does come with a few potential long-term complications. But fear not, my friend, for knowledge is power!

One of the most common long-term complications is vitamin and nutrient deficiencies. Yep, those sneaky little nutrients might try to play hide-and-seek with you. But fret not! With proper guidance from your healthcare team, you can keep those nutrients in check with supplements and a well-balanced diet. You will be on lifelong multi vitamin, calcium, and iron supplements to prevent those deficiencies. Check DoctorKudsi.com for a list of vitamins that could help prevent nutrient deficiencies.

Another potential issue is gastroesophageal reflux disease (GERD). It's like your stomach decides to become a bit of a troublemaker, sending acid up your esophagus uninvited. The good news is there are ways to manage this villainous reflux. Medications, lifestyle adjustments, and even some superfoods that soothe the tummy can come to your rescue. If GERD is not manageable with lifestyle changes and medications, some people may need a revisional surgery to help control the symptoms. As discussed previously gastric bypass would be the most common option.

Let's not forget about the possibility of strictures, which involves narrowing of the stomach. Usually this could happen the first few weeks after surgery. If you encounter this pesky situation, there are techniques like balloon dilations to help widen things up and get you back on track.

And of course, weight regain might try to sneak its way into the picture. It's like those extra pounds are plotting a comeback! Remember, sleeve gastrectomy is a team effort, and with support from your healthcare team, healthy lifestyle choices, and a dose of determination, you can keep those pounds from knocking on your door.

37. Will I experience any changes in my bowel movements after sleeve gastrectomy?

After a sleeve gastrectomy, your digestive system might decide to do some acrobatics. Think of it like a Cirque du Soleil performance in your belly!

While this procedure does wonders for your waistline, it can also have some unexpected effects on your bathroom routine. So, let's dive into the world of post-surgery bowel movements!

First off, say goodbye to those monstrous, Godzilla-sized meals you used to devour. Your stomach has shrunk, my friend, so your food intake will be significantly smaller. With less food going in, you can expect a reduced output on the other end.

Now, let's talk speed. With a smaller stomach, your food will zip through your digestive system faster than a cheetah on roller skates. That means you might find yourself dashing to the restroom from time to time. Just make sure you don't trip on your shoelaces while sprinting, okay?

And let's not forget about the quality of your bowel movements. Since you'll be eating less and your body is adapting to the changes, you might notice some alterations in texture and consistency. Your poop might become more compact and drier than before.

Don't get too concerned though. These changes are all part of the adjustment process. Your body is simply adapting to the new normal after the sleeve gastrectomy. To get your bowel movements back on track, try upping your fiber and water game, or maybe give over-the-counter stuff like fiber supplements, stool softeners, or laxatives a shot.

38. Can sleeve gastrectomy cause dumping syndrome?

Ah, the curious case of sleeve gastrectomy and the infamous dumping syndrome.

Dumping syndrome occurs when food makes a swift exit from your stomach into the small intestine without following the proper traffic rules. Usually, it comes with its own set of "side effects" that can leave you feeling a little off-kilter. It can involve bloating, abdominal cramps, sweating, and a sudden urge to find the nearest restroom.

But fear not, because dumping syndrome can serve as a friendly reminder to approach your meals with caution. It's like a mischievous friend nudging you and saying, "Hey, slow down there, buddy! Let's savor the flavors and enjoy the journey together!"

Here's the scoop: Sleeve gastrectomy can indeed increase the likelihood of experiencing dumping syndrome, especially if you indulge in sugary or fatty treats or rush through your meals. It's like a stern reminder to make mindful choices and listen to your body's cues.

The good news is dumping syndrome is usually temporary and can be managed with some clever strategies. Embrace the art of portion control, choose nutrient-dense foods, and savor each bite like a food connoisseur. It's like turning your mealtime intc a food appreciation show, complete with slow-motion chewing and exaggerated enjoyment!

Now, it's essential to remember that not everyone who undergoes sleeve gastrectomy experiences dumping syndrome. In fact, most people do not! It's like a surprise guest who may or may not show up to your post-meal party. But if they do, rest assured that with time, you'll learn to navigate this quirky aspect of your weight loss journey.

39. Can sleeve gastrectomy lead to hair loss?

Alright, let's tackle the hairy topic of hair loss after sleeve gastrectomy.

Imagine you're in a hair salon, ready for a style transformation after sleeve gastrectomy. But wait, there's a twist! Along with the pounds, you might notice your luscious locks taking a vacation, too. Don't worry, my friend; it's just a temporary break—they'll be back!

Here's the scoop: Sleeve gastrectomy can occasionally lead to hair loss!

So, why does this happen? Well, after sleeve gastrectomy, your body goes through some pretty amazing changes. Rapid weight loss, changes in nutrition, and shifts in hormone levels can all contribute to hair loss. It's like a temporary side effect, a blip on the radar of your weight loss journey.

But, here's the good news! Hair loss after sleeve gastrectomy is usually temporary and self-limiting. In most cases, your hair will start growing back within a few months, just like a lush garden sprouting in springtime!

In the meantime, you might want to embrace your inner rock star and experiment with different hairstyles or rock some fabulous headscarves. Think of it as a chance to explore new looks and unleash your inner fashionista!

To minimize hair loss, first and foremost, let's talk protein, the superhero nutrient that will fuel your body's transformation. Aim to consume a minimum of 60 to 80 grams of protein each day. It's like building a protein fortress to keep your body strong and ready for any challenge! Make protein your trusty sidekick by including it in every meal—breakfast, lunch, dinner, and even those epic snack moments. Protein shakes, eggs, lean meats, Greek yogurt, and legumes are all fantastic choices that will add to your protein count!

Sometimes, though, your protein might require a little boost. Enter liquid or powdered protein supplements, your secret weapons for meeting your daily protein goals. Just mix them up with your favorite beverage, and voila! You've got a protein-packed potion to keep you on track.

Now, let's sprinkle some vitamins and minerals into the mix. Some of the vitamins and minerals that are essential to minimize hair loss include:

- Biotin: Biotin-rich foods include eggs, almonds, cauliflower, cheese, mushrooms, sweet potato, and spinach.

- Iron: Iron-rich foods include lean meats, seafood, beans, dark leafy vegetables, and fortified grains.

- Vitamin D: Some studies suggest that vitamin D may help activate hair growth. It's found in fatty fish, cheese, and egg yolks, and your body also produces it in response to sunlight.

- Zinc: Plays an important role in hair tissue growth and repair. Foods high in zinc include oysters, beef, spinach, wheat germ, pumpkin seeds, and lentils.

Remember, my friend, hair loss after sleeve gastrectomy is a temporary detour on your weight loss adventure. It's like a pit stop for your hair follicles to catch their breath before they come back stronger and more fabulous than ever!

40. Will I need to follow a special diet after sleeve gastrectomy?

Get ready to dive into the world of pre- and post-surgery diets, folks! It's like a culinary adventure with twists and turns that will make your taste buds go wild. So, grab your forks and let's dig into the highlights of this special diet!

First things first, we have the phases of the diet. It's like leveling up in a video game, but instead of unlocking new abilities, you're unlocking different food textures and consistencies. You start with clear liquids, move on to full liquids, pureed foods, soft foods, and finally, you conquer the ultimate challenge—a regular solid food diet. You'll go from sipping on broths to conquering a steak with your trusty knife and fork! Your surgeon will use his own protocol to advance your diet. For my own post op nutrition plan check my website DoctorKudsi.com

Portion control is the name of the game when you have a smaller stomach. It's like being a master of mini meals, where you eat smaller portions throughout the day. And remember, listening to your body's signals of hunger and fullness is crucial. You'll now have a built-in food alarm system that tells you when it's time to chow down or when to put down the fork and call it a day.

Now, let's talk about the art of slow eating and chewing. It's like attending a gourmet feast where you savor every bite like a true food connoisseur. Taking your time to chew your food thoroughly not only prevents discomfort but also gives your body a chance to properly digest those culinary masterpieces. Bon appétit, my friend!

When it comes to the special diet, nutrient-dense foods take the center stage. Think of each meal like a show with a cast of superstars consisting of lean proteins, fruits, vegetables, whole grains, and healthy fats. These culinary superheroes provide essential nutrients while keeping your calorie intake in check. Think of them as the Avengers of the food world, keeping your body strong and healthy!

Hydration is key, my friends! It's like fueling up your body with liquid awesomeness. But remember, the hydration game has rules—drink plenty of fluids between meals but avoid chugging during your munching sessions. We don't want to flood that precious stomach of yours. And hey, water is the MVP in the hydration squad, so drink up!

Now, let's address the troublemakers—the problematic foods. Consider them a group of rebellious ingredients that can cause discomfort or digestive issues. We're talking about high-fat or greasy foods, carbonated beverages (no fizzy party in your tummy), tough meats that put your chewing skills to the test, fibrous veggies that require a little extra TLC, and the sugary or high-calorie treats that are just too tempting to resist. It's like avoiding a minefield of culinary chaos!

Last, but not least, with reduced food intake, you'll need these lifelong vitamin supplements to prevent deficiencies. It's like having your own team of tiny capsules, providing you with all the essential nutrients like B12, iron, calcium, and more. These bariatric vitamins are like superheroes in pill form, ensuring your body gets everything it needs to stay healthy.

So, there you have it—all the deets on your new special diet extravaganza. Embrace the adventure, savor each bite, and remember to laugh along the way. You're on a culinary quest like no other, and with the right mindset, you'll conquer it all!

41. How important is water after sleeve gastrectomy?

Let me emphasize the importance of the most important glorious task after your surgery. Listen up because it's time for a hydration crash course!

Your main full-time job post-surgery is none other than drinking. Yes, you heard it right! Your trusty water bottle becomes your loyal companion, and sipping becomes your ultimate mission. Forget about solving complex equations or climbing Mount Everest—hydration takes the crown!

Why is it so crucial? Well, imagine the horror of ending up dehydrated and getting a one-way ticket back to the hospital. Trust me, that's not the kind of adventure you signed up for! Staying hydrated is key to your recovery and overall well-being.

So, let's make a pact, shall we? Promise yourself to be the hydration champion. Keep that water bottle by your side like a loyal sidekick. Sip, gulp, and chug throughout the day.

I am kidding! No gulping and chugging—only sipping!

Don't let thirst sneak up on you. Stay one step ahead and hydrate!

Remember, water is your secret weapon against dehydration. And if you want to add some zest to your hydration routine, feel free to infuse your water with slices of citrus, refreshing mint, or whatever floats your boat. Get creative and make hydration your happy habit!

42. Will I need to take vitamin and mineral supplements after the sleeve gastrectomy?

Alright, let's talk about the supplement party after sleeve gastrectomy! It's like a nutritional extravaganza with vitamins and minerals taking the spotlight. So, get ready to pop those supplement bottles!

First up, we have multivitamins comprised of essential nutrients, fighting for your overall health. Think of them as your personal squad of miniature superheroes, packed with vitamins and minerals to keep you thriving. Just make sure to choose the bariatric vitamin brands that follow the ASMBS (American Society for Metabolic and Bariatric Surgery) guidelines because we don't want any rogue superheroes causing trouble!

Next on the list, we have the dynamic duo—calcium and vitamin D. They're like the Batman and Robin of bone health, ensuring your skeleton stays strong and your teeth stay pearly white. With the reduced stomach size, these supplements swoop in to save the day and make sure your bones can handle any dance move or silly slip-up.

An iron supplement is also key, preventing or treating iron deficiency anemia. After weight loss surgery, it's important to keep those iron levels in check and avoid any fatigue. So, embrace the iron supplement and unleash your increased energy! The amount of iron you should take can change depending on factors like your age and gender. So, it's a good idea to chat with your own surgeon to figure out the right amount for you.

And hey, don't forget to keep up with your regular catch-ups with your healthcare crew. They're ace at working out the best mix and timing for your supplements so they don't mess with any meds you're on. Plus, they're on point with making sure you're not short on any nutrients. So, give it some attention, your health's worth it!

Remember, after sleeve gastrectomy, the supplement game is key to helping you enjoy your new, healthier you!

43. Will I need to make permanent changes to my eating habits after sleeve gastrectomy?

Brace yourself for a delicious truth: Yes, you'll need to make some changes to your eating habits. But fear not! It's not as dreadful as it sounds. In fact, think of it as a culinary adventure, a chance to explore new flavors and embrace a healthier lifestyle.

Imagine your pre-surgery eating habits as a wild carnival ride, full of ups, downs, and twists. Well, after the sleeve gastrectomy, you're hopping onto a gentler carousel, where portion control and mindful eating take center stage.

You see, your stomach is now smaller and more selective about its guests. It can't handle those gargantuan portions you once devoured. But fret not, my friend, because this simply means you get to savor every bite, transforming each meal into a delectable experience.

Now, let's talk about the foods you'll want to prioritize. Think protein, my pal! Fill your plate with lean meats, fish, eggs, and legumes, which will keep you satisfied and help your body recover. Oh, and don't forget about those colorful veggies and fruits, bursting with vitamins and nutrients to fuel your superhero self.

But hey, we're only human, and cravings will still knock on your door like an enthusiastic neighbor. It's okay to indulge in small amounts of your favorite treats occasionally. Just remember to savor them, enjoy every morsel, and practice moderation like a master.

Oh, and here's a little tip: chewing your food thoroughly and taking your time during meals is not only good manners but also beneficial for digestion. It's like giving a slow clap to your taste buds!

Now, here's a quick summary -

– Eat three meals each day

– Chew your food thoroughly

– Start each meal with a protein source

– Stop eating just before you feel full.

– Drink between each meal, not with your meals

– Keep unhealthy foods out of the house

– Don't eat in front of the TV as you might overeat

And last but not least – Don't go to the grocery store hungry!

Hunger and grocery shopping are a bad combination.

So, my foodie friend, while some changes are in store for your eating habits, they're not a life sentence of blandness. Embrace this culinary adventure with open arms, discover new recipes, and create a harmonious dance between your taste buds and your newfound healthy lifestyle.

Remember, food is meant to be enjoyed, and with your sleeve gastrectomy as your trusty guide, you're on the path to slimming success, one delicious bite at a time! Bon appétit!

44. Will I be able to eat normal-sized meals after sleeve gastrectomy?

Picture this: You, a post-surgery foodie, standing at the crossroads of portion sizes, wondering if "normal" meals will still have a place on your plate. Well, my friend, prepare for a culinary adventure that will have you questioning the definition of "normal."

Here's the scoop: After your sleeve gastrectomy, your stomach undergoes a bit of a makeover. It transforms into a svelte and sleek portion controller. But fear not, brave eater, for "normal" is a relative term. Your new normal will be a bit different from your pre-surgery normal. You may find that your stomach's capacity has decreased, and it's more like a cozy bistro rather than an all-you-can-eat buffet.

So, yes, you can still enjoy meals, just in smaller portions. It's like downsizing from a super-sized meal to a charming tapas feast. Quality over quantity! So put on your food detective hat and explore new ways to make your meals exciting and delicious. Get creative with flavors, textures, and spices to jazz up those smaller portions. Your taste buds will be grateful for the flavorful adventures.

45. Can I drink alcohol after sleeve gastrectomy?

Now, picture this: You, post-surgery, again! standing at another crossroads this time of fun and responsibility, wondering if alcohol is still on the menu. Well, my friend, the answer isn't as clear as vodka on the rocks. But fear not, for I shall serve up some knowledge.

The short answer is that you should not drink alcohol for one year after your surgery. Now, here comes the funny part: Your new stomach size might turn into a bit of a party pooper. This means that alcohol might affect you differently than before. So, after surgery alcohol can pack a punch in smaller quantities. That means you might feel the effects quicker than a tipsy cheetah on roller skates. So, caution and moderation become your trusty drinking buddies.

Also, keep in mind that alcohol isn't exactly a nutritious smoothie. It's high in calories and low in nutritional value. So, while a little indulgence now and then might not hurt, it's important to balance it with a healthy diet and lifestyle.

Now, let's talk hydration. Alcohol can be a sneaky dehydrator, leaving you feeling as parched as a cactus in the desert. And hey, hydration is key to staying healthy and feeling your best! So, make sure to sip on that H2O like it's the elixir of life alongside any adult beverages you choose to enjoy.

But hey, there's also a world of delicious mocktails, creative concoctions, and refreshing alternatives to explore. After all, who needs alcohol when you can sip on a mocktail masterpiece that leaves your taste buds dancing? And here is another reminder to avoid carbonated drinks the first few months after surgery!

So, my beverage enthusiast, whether you choose to imbibe or opt for the mocktail extravaganza, remember to sip wisely, hydrate like a boss, and let the post-surgery adventures continue with an occasional clink of glasses! Cheers to your health and happiness!

46. How soon after sleeve gastrectomy can I start exercising?

Well, look at you, Mr./Ms. Early Bird, already thinking about exercising after sleeve gastrectomy! That's a fantastic sign that you're on the path to lifelong success! But hold your horses, or should I say, dumbbells. Let's dive into the world of post-surgery exercise!

On the night of your surgery, get ready to strut your stuff like a model on a catwalk. You'll be walking as much as you want, flaunting your hospital gown like it's a designer outfit. And don't forget to show off your stair-climbing skills because you'll be going up and down those steps like a champ. Who needs an elevator when you've got newly found surgical superpowers, right?

But wait, there's a little weightlifting disclaimer. For the first few weeks, leave the heavy lifting to the professionals. No, I'm not talking about bodybuilders or wrestlers. I'm talking about lifting more than 10-15lbs. So, put down those heavy dumbbells and embrace the lighter side of life. It's like a temporary ban on heavy lifting, giving your body the chance to heal and adjust to its new sleeve status.

Now, mark your calendars for the grand return of physical activity in 4-6 weeks. It's like waiting for the release of your favorite movie—exciting and full of anticipation. Once that magical time arrives, you can unleash your inner exercise enthusiast and do any physical activity your heart desires. Whether it's jogging, yoga, or even attempting to break the world record for the most enthusiastic jumping jacks, the choice is yours. So, get ready to break free and conquer the fitness world!

Oh, and if you're craving a week-by-week exercise regimen, check out the appendices of this book or my website DoctorKudsi.com too if you need help to find the perfect workout for each week. And be sure to choose an activity that's fun for you. Get ready to sweat, laugh, and enjoy the journey to lifelong success!

So, embrace your early exercise enthusiasm, but don't forget to give your body the time it needs to recover. Soon enough, you'll be back in action, conquering the world one workout at a time.

47. Can I get pregnant after sleeve gastrectomy?

Guess what? The sleeve gastrectomy isn't just a weight-loss hero—it can be a help to fertility, too! That's right, ladies, you can still rock that baby bump after the sleeve gastrectomy. In fact, this surgery can boost your chances of getting pregnant and give you a healthier pregnancy.

For many, weight loss leads to improved fertility. It's like shedding those extra pounds and finding the secret recipe for baby-making success. Say goodbye to fertility struggles caused by obesity and hello to a higher chance of conceiving.

But wait, there's more! With sleeve gastrectomy, you get reduced risks of pregnancy complications. Meaning less chance of having gestational diabetes, high blood pressure, and other pesky problems. Pregnancy can be an exciting time, but it also comes with some worries. Having your weight under control can help alleviate some of those worries!

And hey, if you had pre-existing conditions like type 2 diabetes or sleep apnea, sleeve gastrectomy comes to the rescue! Better control of those conditions means fewer risks during pregnancy.

But wait, there's a bonus! Losing excess weight can improve your mobility and comfort during pregnancy. It's like shedding those pounds and gaining the ability to move like a graceful gazelle. You've set yourself up for a smoother pregnancy experience in many ways.

So, overall sleeve gastrectomy is like a fertility booster, a complication reducer, and a superhero sidekick for your health. Get ready to rock that baby bump and laugh in the face of pregnancy challenges. You've got this, supermom-to-be! Now the final reminder. Sleeve gastrectomy can lead to nutritional deficiencies which might impact fetal development. So, remember to take your vitamins and follow regularly with your healthcare team.

48. What should I do if I'm not losing weight as expected after sleeve gastrectomy?

Oh, dear weight loss warrior, if the scale isn't budging as much as expected after your sleeve gastrectomy, fear not! We've got some tricks up our sleeve to get that weight loss train chugging along. So, grab a seat and let's dive into the action plan!

First things first, take a deep breath and remember that weight loss journeys can be as unpredictable as the weather. Sometimes, our bodies decide to do their own funky dance moves, and the weight loss takes a detour. But hey, no worries! Here are a few tips to get back on track.

Revisit Your Eating Habits: Double-check your eating habits and make sure you're following the post-op guidelines to the tee. Are you savoring those small, nutritious meals? Are you taking your time, chewing your food thoroughly, and listening to your body's signals?

Hello, Hydration: Hydration is the name of the game! Make sure you're sipping on that water like it's your favorite summer beverage. Staying hydrated not only keeps you feeling refreshed but can also help with weight loss. It's like giving your body a big, cool high-five!

Get Moving and Grooving: Time to shake that body and get those limbs moving! Regular physical activity can give your weight loss journey an extra boost. So, find an activity you enjoy, whether it's dancing like nobody's watching or taking scenic walks in the park. It's like throwing a party for your body and saying, "Let's burn some calories and have a blast!" Remember, stick to my post op exercise plan at the end of the book! Anything less than one hour a day of structured exercising will not help with weight loss. Those are the studies talking, not me!

Seek Support: Remember, you're not alone in this adventure! Reach out to your healthcare team, your trusty group of weight loss cheerleaders. They can offer guidance, evaluate your progress, and provide personalized tips to help you get back on the weight loss wagon. They might even prescribe you some weight loss medications that will help give you the extra nudge you need.

Patience, Grasshopper: Rome wasn't built in a day, and neither will your dream body. Weight loss is a journey, and it takes time for those pounds to bid farewell. Don't get discouraged if the numbers on the scale aren't dropping as fast as you'd like. Trust the process, stay positive, and celebrate those non-scale victories along the way. It's like giving yourself a big high-five and saying, "I'm making progress, one step at a time!"

Remember, my friend, your sleeve gastrectomy is a tool on your weight loss adventure. Sometimes, the tool needs a little nudge or a tweak, but with a positive attitude and some adjustments, you'll be back on track before you know it. So, keep that chin up, keep believing in yourself, and keep pushing forward. You've got this, weight loss warrior!

49. What should I do if I experience excessive loose skin after sleeve gastrectomy?

Now, after sleeve gastrectomy, it's true that some people may experience loose skin as they bid farewell to those extra pounds. It's like your skin went on a vacation and forgot to pack its elastic band!

But fear not, for there are a few options at your disposal to deal with this flappy situation. First off, give your skin some time to do its magic. Sometimes, it just needs a little bit of time to adjust and tighten up. Also embrace the power of exercise! Regular physical activity, like strength training and toning exercises, can help tighten up those loose areas and give your skin a little boost.

Another trick up our sleeve is hydration! Keep your skin happy and healthy by drinking plenty of water. Hydration helps maintain skin elasticity and keeps it looking fabulous. Plus, it's good for your overall wellbeing too!

Now, if the loose skin is causing you serious frustration, you can always explore cosmetic procedures. Yeah, we're talking about plastic surgery! Procedures like tummy tucks or body lifts can help remove excess skin and give you that smooth, sleek appearance you've been dreaming of. It's like saying, "Goodbye, loose skin! Hello, fabulousness!"

So, whether you decide to let time work its magic, unleash the power of exercise, or opt for a little surgical assistance, remember that loose skin doesn't have to rain on your parade. You've come a long way on your weight loss journey, and loose skin is just a battle scar that tells the world, "Hey, I fought the weight loss battle and won!"

Keep rocking that newfound confidence, my friend, and let loose skin be your reminder of the amazing transformation you've achieved!

50. Will I need to undergo body contouring surgery after significant weight loss from sleeve gastrectomy?

After shedding those pounds with the help of sleeve gastrectomy, you might be wondering if it's time for a grand finale with body contouring surgery.

Now, after achieving significant weight loss, it's like you've become the main character in your very own makeover montage. Sleeve gastrectomy sets the stage by kick-starting your weight loss journey, but the final act—body contouring surgery—is like the grand finale, adding those finishing touches to your transformed physique.

You see, as you drop those pounds, your skin might start, feeling a bit loose and jiggly. Body contouring surgery steps in like a skilled tailor, snipping and tucking to help you achieve a more sculpted appearance. It's like ordering a custom-fitted suit that accentuates your new, fabulous figure!

Now body contouring surgery isn't always a requirement. It's like an optional bonus track on your weight loss album. While it can help address excess skin and improve body proportions, not everyone feels the need for this encore performance.

Factors like age, genetics, and the amount of weight loss can influence whether body contouring surgery becomes a part of your transformation story. It's a personal decision that you'll make in consultation with your healthcare team, considering your goals and desires.

But fear not; even if body contouring surgery isn't in the script, there are other ways to embrace your new body and rock it like a superstar! Embrace your uniqueness, celebrate your achievements, and remember that confidence is the best outfit you can wear.

And hey, don't forget to give yourself a standing ovation for the incredible journey you've embarked upon. Whether you choose body contouring or not, you've already achieved something remarkable with sleeve gastrectomy. You've taken control of your health and rewritten your story with laughter, determination, and a touch of magic!

Conclusion

In conclusion, Sleeve Gastrectomy Surgery Unleashed: Your Witty Q&A Guide to Slimming Success is more than just a book; it is a beacon of motivation and empowerment for those embarking on a transformative journey toward a healthier and happier life.

Through the pages of this book, we have explored the ins and outs of sleeve gastrectomy surgery, demystifying the process and equipping you with the knowledge and tools necessary for success. But beyond the technicalities, we have delved into the depths of your innermost questions, providing witty and insightful answers that will keep you engaged and motivated throughout your slimming journey.

Remember, this is not just a surgical procedure but a catalyst for a life-changing transformation. It is a commitment to yourself, an investment in your wellbeing, and a testament to your strength and determination. As you navigate the challenges and triumphs that lie ahead, always keep in mind the power within you to achieve lasting success.

Embrace the journey with a sense of curiosity, resilience, and a dash of humor. Celebrate every milestone, no matter how small, and learn from every setback. Surround yourself with a support network of loved ones, healthcare professionals, and fellow travelers who will lift you up when you need it most.

Know that you have the ability to create a new chapter in your life, one that is filled with vitality, confidence, and renewed joy. Let this book serve as your guide, igniting the spark within you to unleash your full potential and embrace the slimmer, healthier version of yourself.

With determination, humor, and unwavering belief, embark on this remarkable journey towards a life transformed. You are capable of achieving the unimaginable, and Sleeve Gastrectomy Surgery Unleashed is here to cheer you on every step of the way.

Your slimming success awaits, so go forth and unleash the extraordinary within you!

Appendices

If you want to know more free resources about bariatric surgery you can check my website DoctorKudsi.com

Dr. Kudsi's Post Bariatric Surgery Exercise Program

Weeks 1-2	- Short walks to promote circulation and prevent blood clots. - Aim for a total of one hour of walking per day.
Weeks 3-4	- Continue with short walks and gradually increase duration and distance. - Incorporate gentle stretching exercises for flexibility.
Weeks 5-6	- Increase the intensity and duration of walks. - Consider low-impact exercises like swimming or stationary cycling.
Weeks 7-8	- Progress walks and consider adding strength training. - Start with light weights or resistance bands, targeting major muscle groups.

Weeks 9-12	- Increase the intensity and duration of cardiovascular exercises (e.g., jogging, cycling, aerobic classes). - Continue strength training, gradually increasing weights or resistance.
Months 3-6	- Continue a combination of cardiovascular exercises, strength training, and flexibility exercises. - Consider working with a personal trainer or attending group exercise classes
Months 6- forever	- Maintain consistency with exercise routine and focus on increasing intensity. - Incorporate higher-intensity exercises like interval training and advanced strength training techniques. - Aim for one hour of structured exercise per day, consisting of 40 minutes of cardio and 20 minutes of strength training.

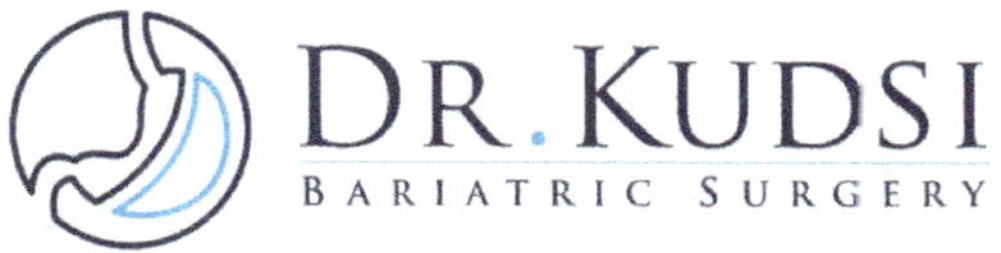

Meet The Author

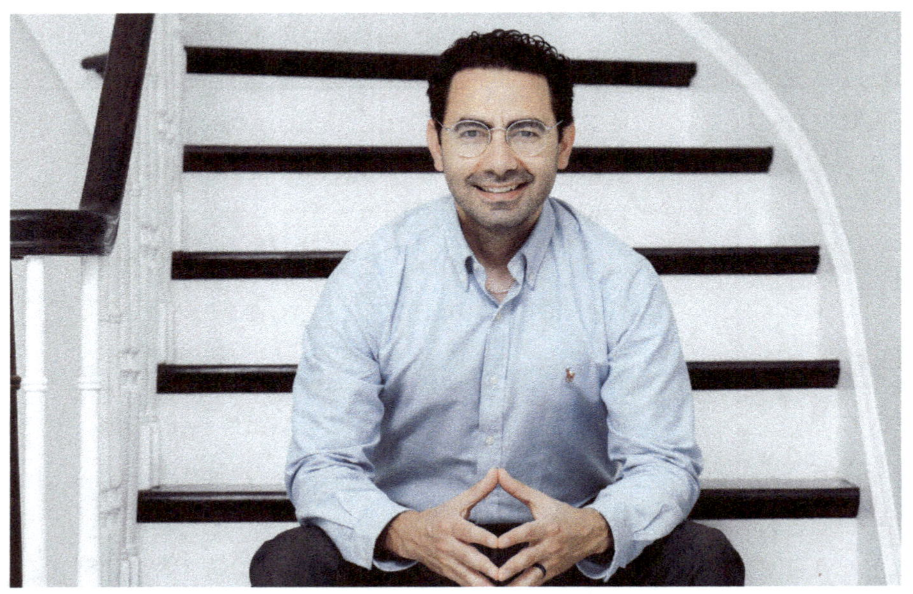

Dr. Jihad Kudsi is a dedicated husband, loving father, and esteemed bariatric surgeon. With a passion for transforming lives through weight loss and improved health, Dr. Kudsi has made significant contributions to the field of bariatric surgery.

Dr. Jihad Kudsi's educational journey has been marked by excellence. He completed his General Surgery Internship at Mayo Clinic in Rochester, MN, and his General Surgery

Residency at George Washington University in Washington, DC. Seeking further expertise, he pursued a fellowship training in Minimally Invasive Surgery/Bariatric Surgery at Houston Methodist Hospital in Houston, TX. Additionally, Dr. Kudsi holds an MBA and Master in Finance from the Indiana University Kelley School of Business, enabling him to bring a unique perspective to his medical practice.

Dr. Jihad Kudsi's dedication to his patients' holistic well-being is mirrored by his dual board certification in General Surgery and Obesity Medicine. He is a recognized Diplomate of the American Board of Obesity Medicine and a proud Fellow of the American College of Surgeons.

Beyond his clinical practice, Dr. Kudsi's influence extends to academia and public education. He authored the "Weight Loss for Life" course, a vital tool for individuals on their path to sustainable weight loss. His commitment to fostering learning and excellence is further reflected in his roles as an Affiliate Clinical Assistant Professor at the University of Dubuque and a spokesperson for The Obesity Society (TOS).

Beyond his clinical practice, Dr. Kudsi holds pivotal leadership positions, serving as the Chair of Surgery at Duly Health and Care and the Medical Director of Bariatric Surgery at the University of Chicago/ LaGrange Hospital in the Chicagoland area. These roles exemplify his authoritative influence and significant responsibilities in overseeing and improving surgical standards and patient outcomes.

Through his expertise, dedication, and compassionate approach to patient care, Dr. Jihad Kudsi has become a trusted leader in the field of bariatric surgery, helping countless individuals achieve their weight loss and wellness goals.

Website: DoctorKudsi.com

Email: DrKudsi@doctorKudsi.com

Facebook: Doctor.Kudsi

Instagram: Doctor.Kudsi

Youtube: Doctor.Kudsi

www.ingramcontent.com/pod-product-compliance
Lightning Source LLC
Chambersburg PA
CBHW070944260726
48661CB00003B/1117

* 9 7 9 8 8 5 8 9 2 0 5 5 7 *